The Cancer Fighting Cookbook

Delicious, Tasty and Stress-Free Recipes to live a Vibrant Lifestyle.

WITH PICTURES

AND

A 7-DAY MEAL PLAN

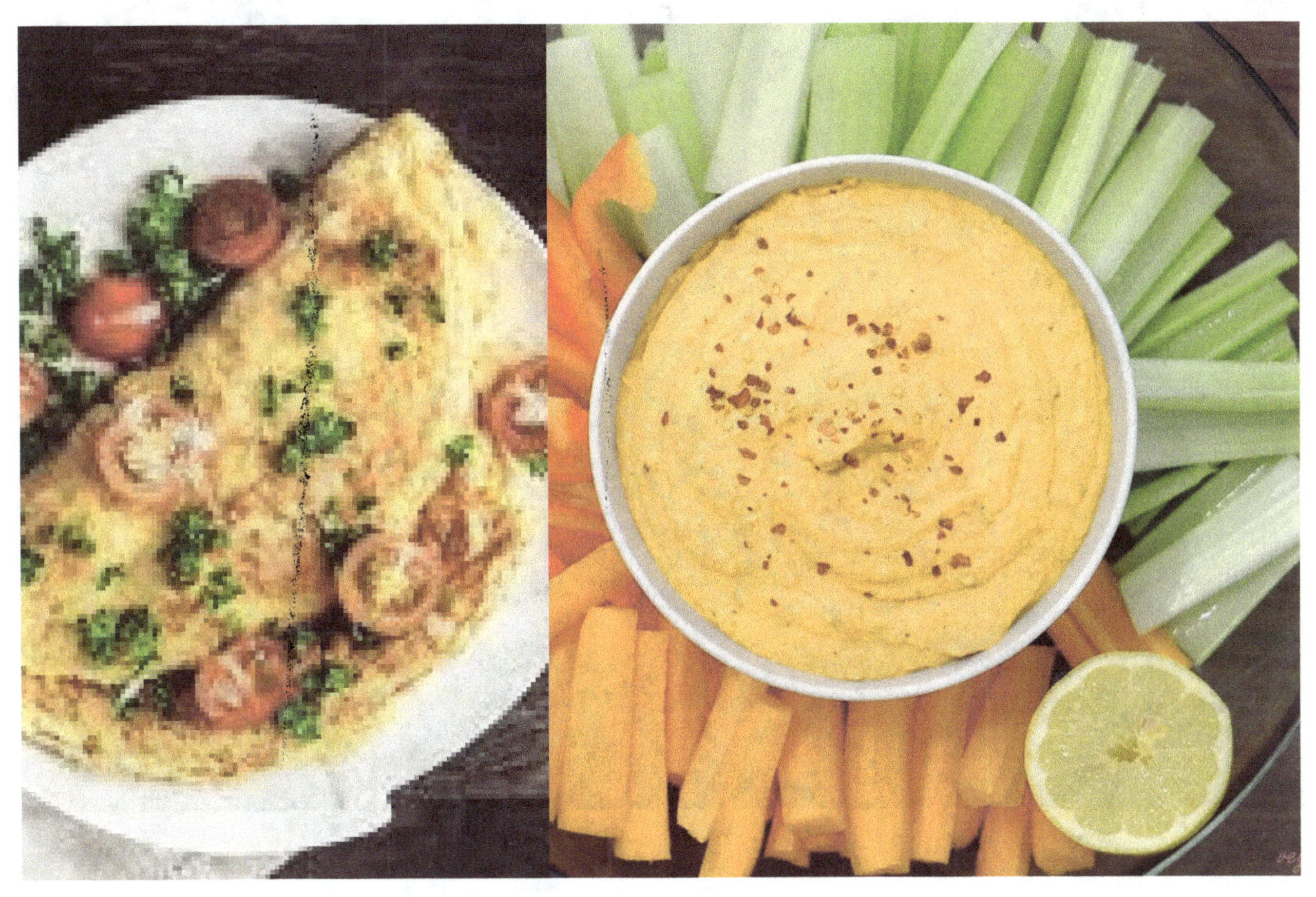

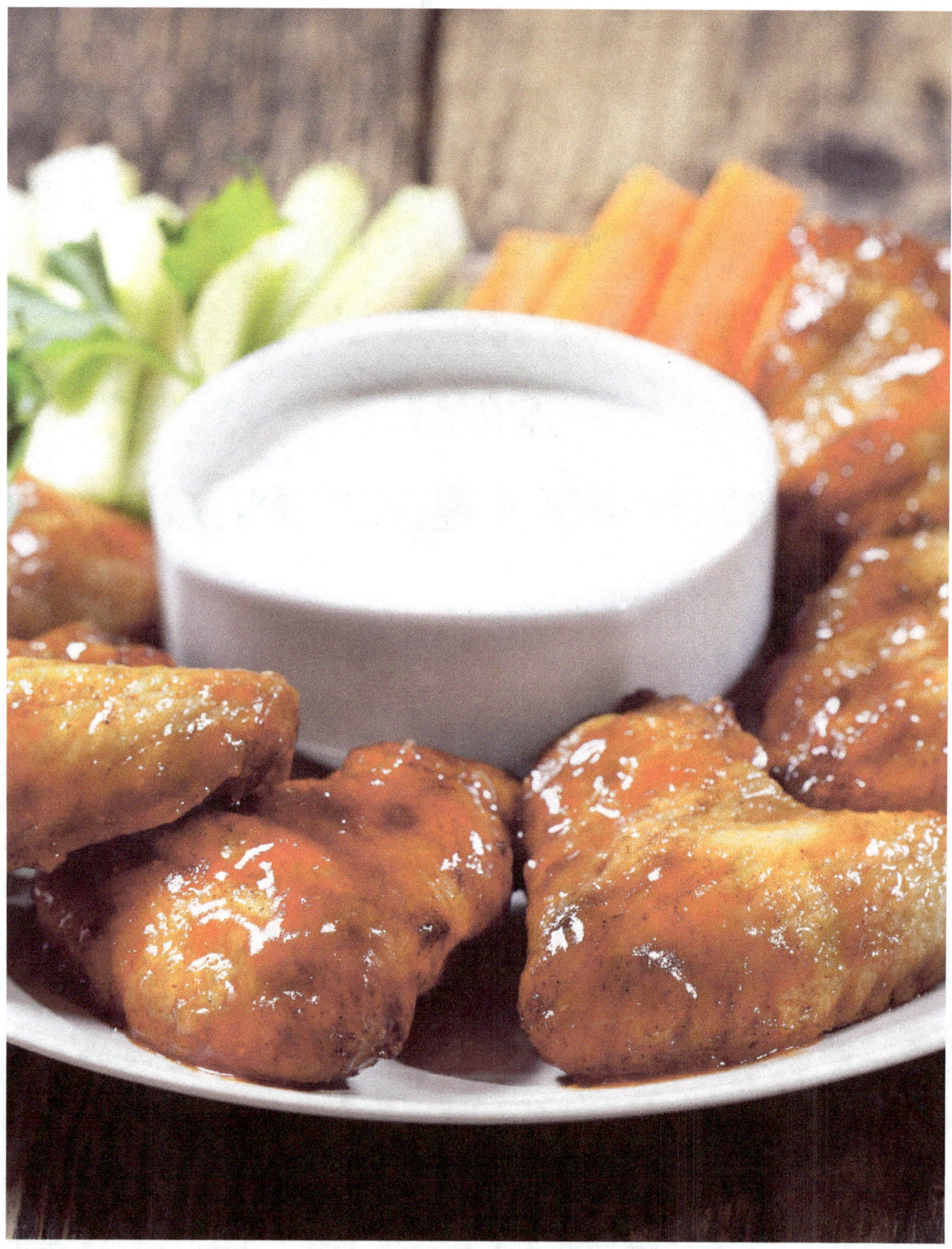

COPYRIGHT PAGE

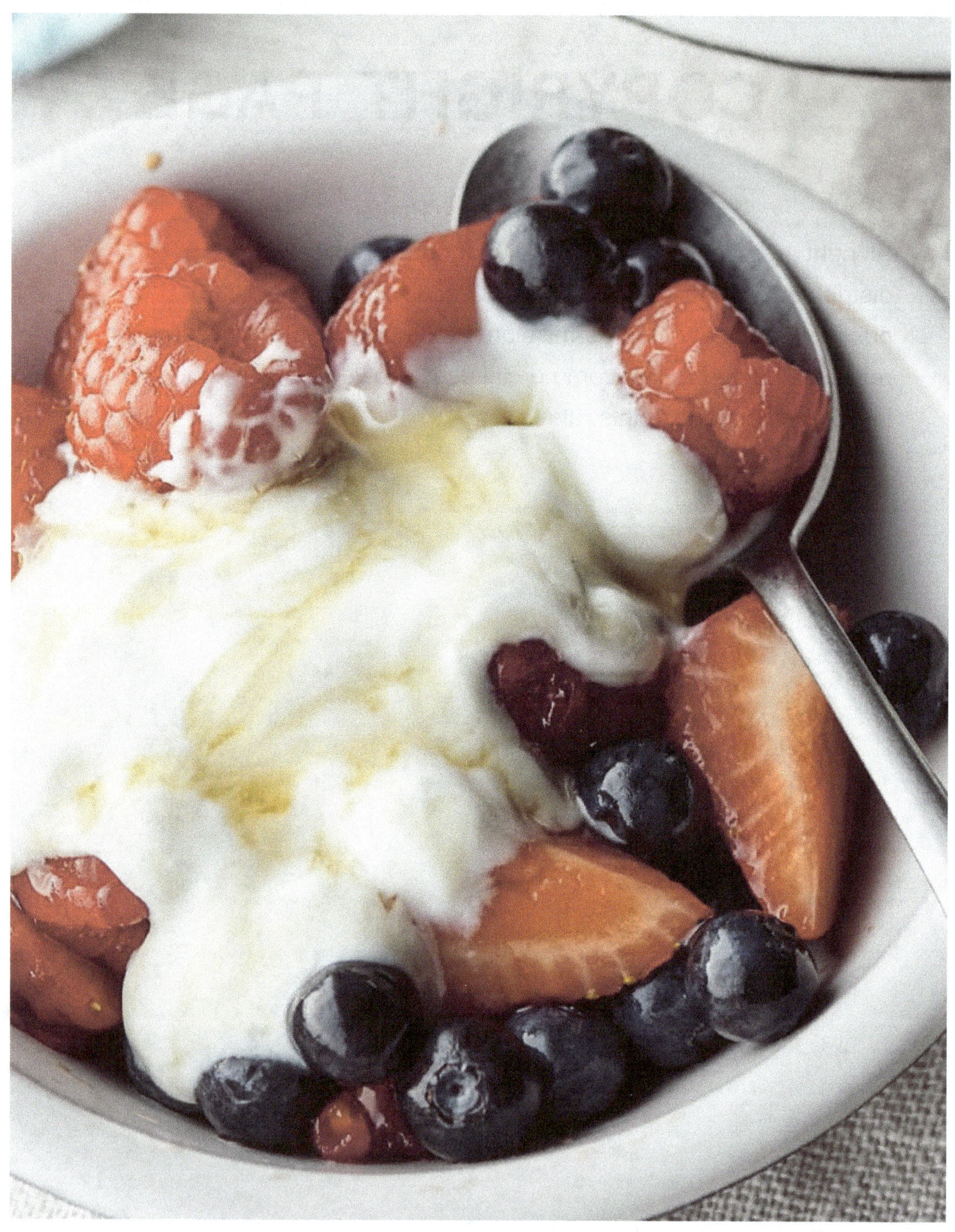

I am deeply grateful to everyone who made "The Cancer Fighting Cookbook: Nourishment for Recovery" possible.

To the medical professionals who generously shared their expertise and insights, thank you for guiding me with your knowledge and experience. To the cancer survivors who bravely shared their stories, your resilience and courage are truly inspiring.

A special thank you to my family and friends for your unwavering support and encouragement. Your love and patience have been my strength throughout this journey.

To my editors, designers, and everyone involved in the production of this book, your hard work and dedication have brought this vision to life.

Lastly, to the readers, thank you for trusting me to be a part of your journey. I hope this book brings you comfort, nourishment, and hope.

With heartfelt gratitude

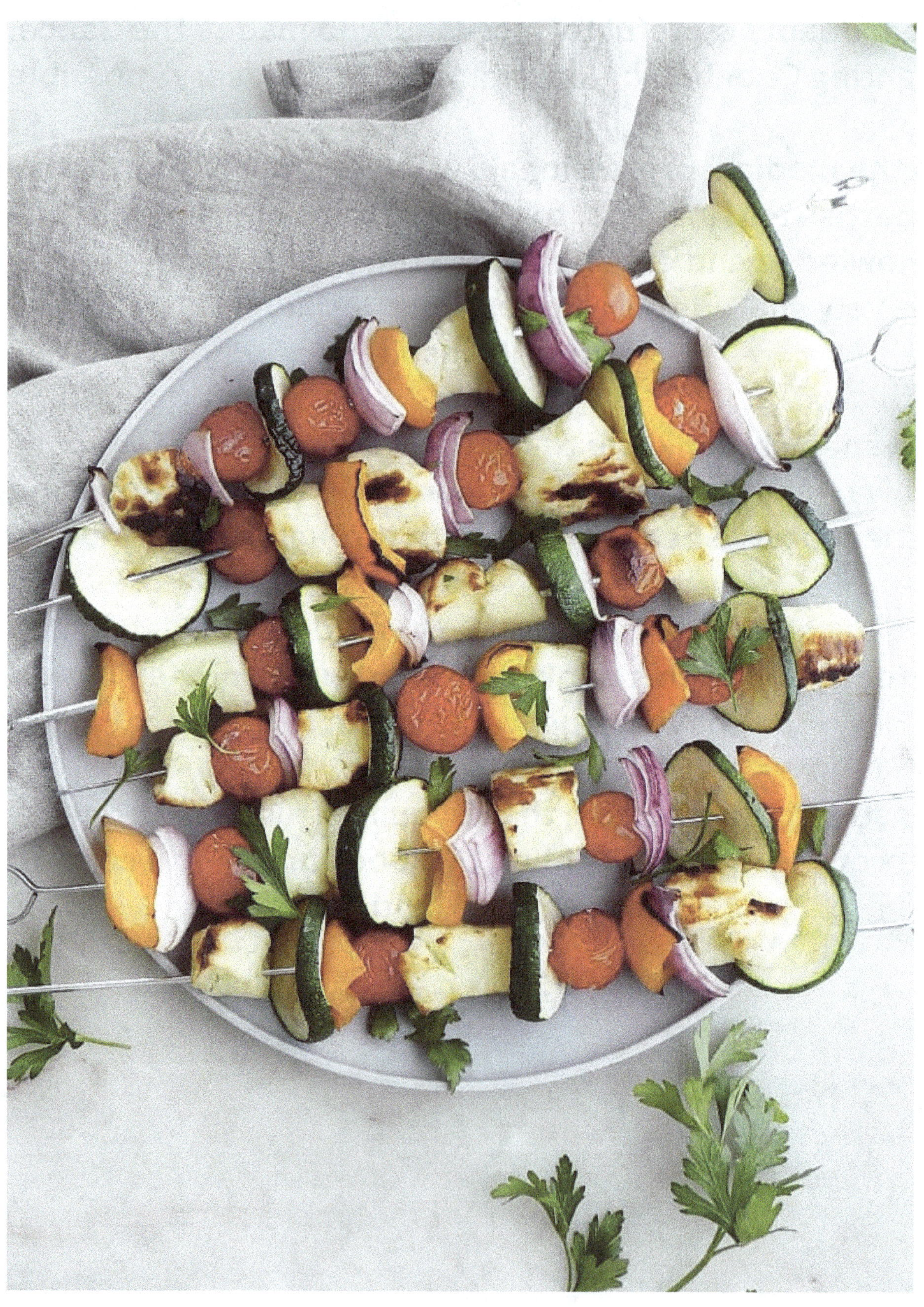

TABLE OF CONTENTS

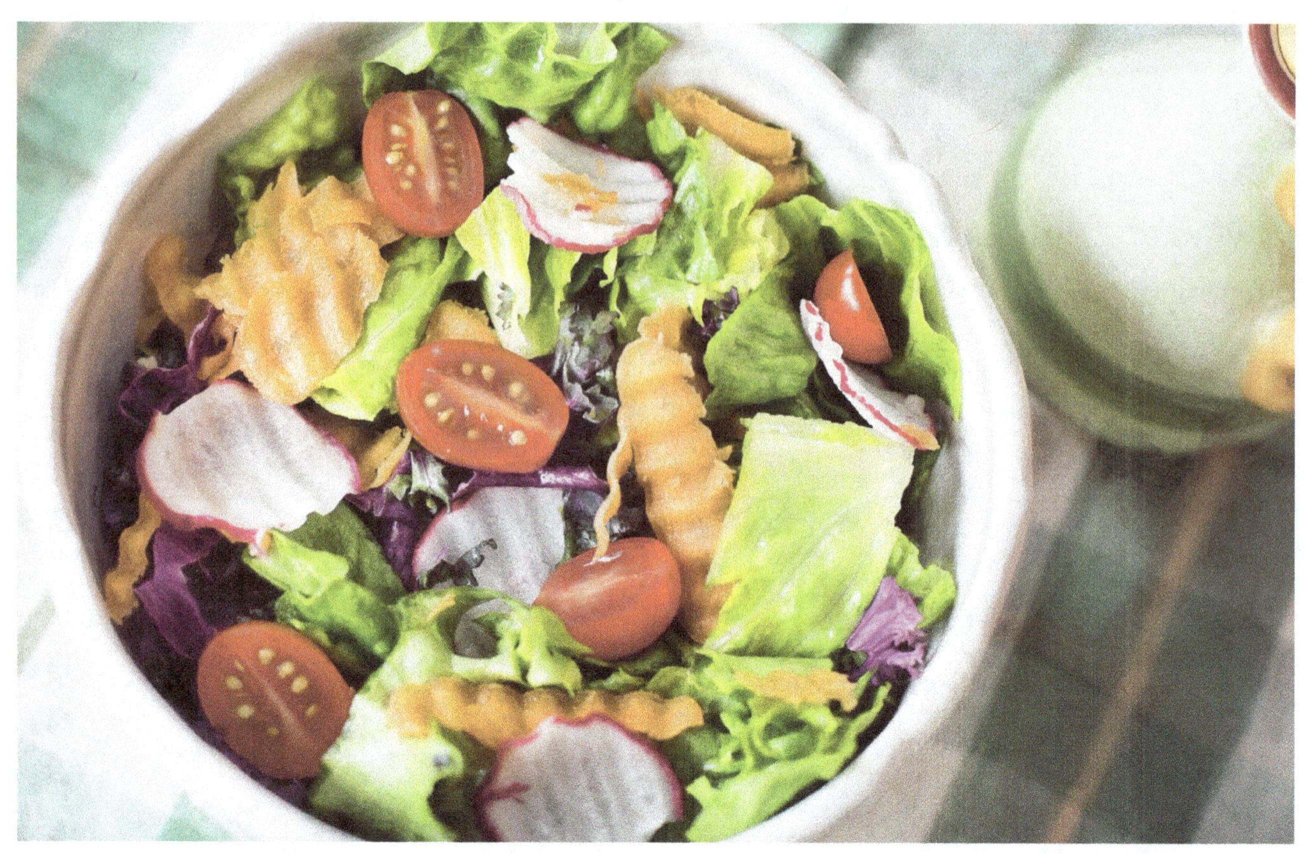

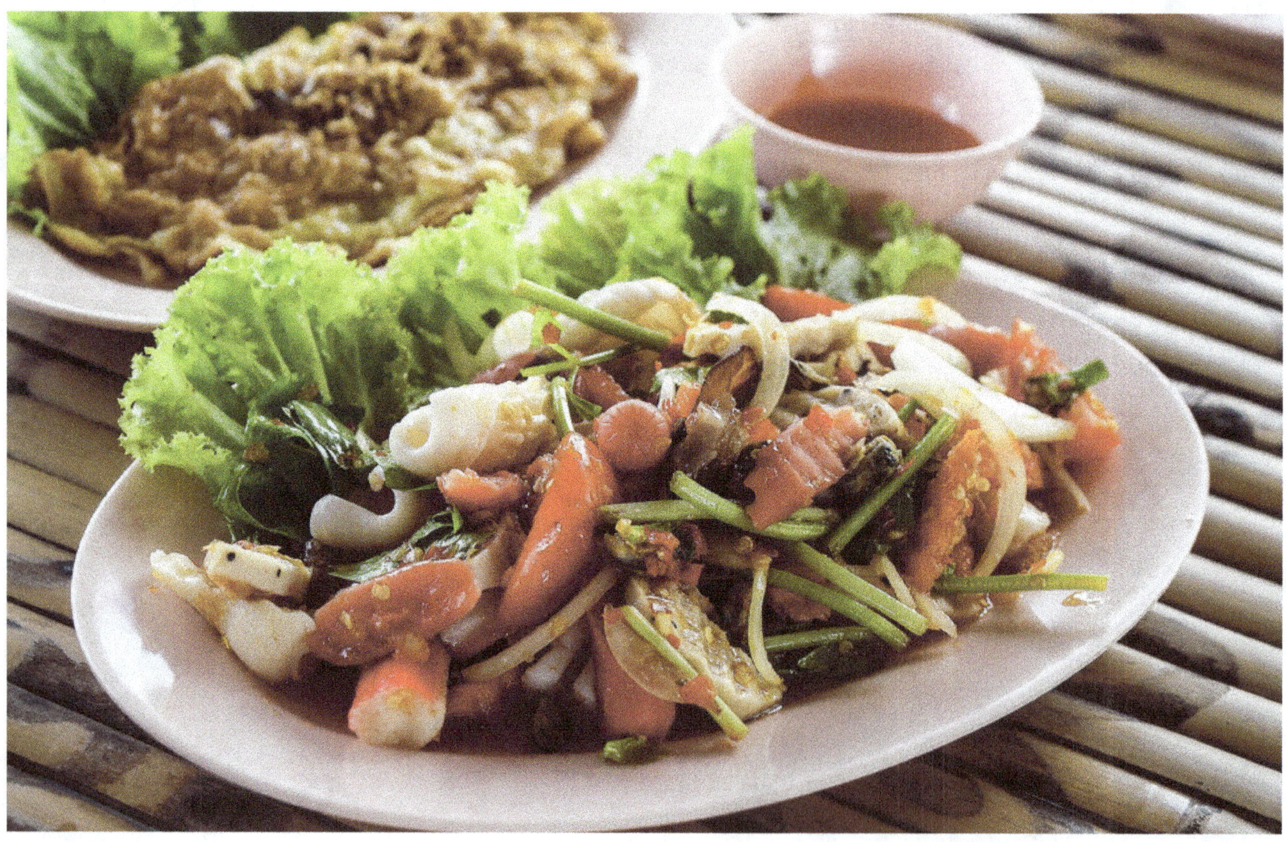

CHAPTER ONE

Understanding Cancer and Nutrition

INTRODUCTION TO CANCER AND IMPACTS OF NUTRITION ON CANCER

Cancer is a diverse category of diseases defined by the uncontrolled development and spread of cells that are abnormal. It can develop in almost any part of the body and has over 100 different types, each with its own set of characteristics and treatment protocols. Common types include lung cancer,breast cancer, prostate cancer, and colorectal cancer. Treatments for cancer vary widely and may include surgery, chemotherapy, radiation therapy, immunotherapy, targeted therapy, and hormone therapy, among others. One of the significant challenges that cancer patients face is maintaining proper nutrition. The disease itself, along with its treatments, can profoundly affect the body's ability to absorb and utilize nutrients. Cancer and its treatments can lead to various side effects such as nausea, vomiting, diarrhea, constipation, loss of appetite, taste changes, and difficulty swallowing. These side effects can hinder a patient's ability to maintain a balanced diet, making nutrition an essential yet challenging component of cancer care. Adequate nutrition is crucial for cancer patients for several reasons. It helps maintain body weight and strength, supports immune function, enhances the effectiveness of treatments, and improves overall quality of life. Good nutrition can help manage treatment side effects, reduce the risk of complications, and promote faster recovery and healing. Therefore, understanding the relationship between cancer and nutrition is vital for patients, caregivers, and healthcare providers.

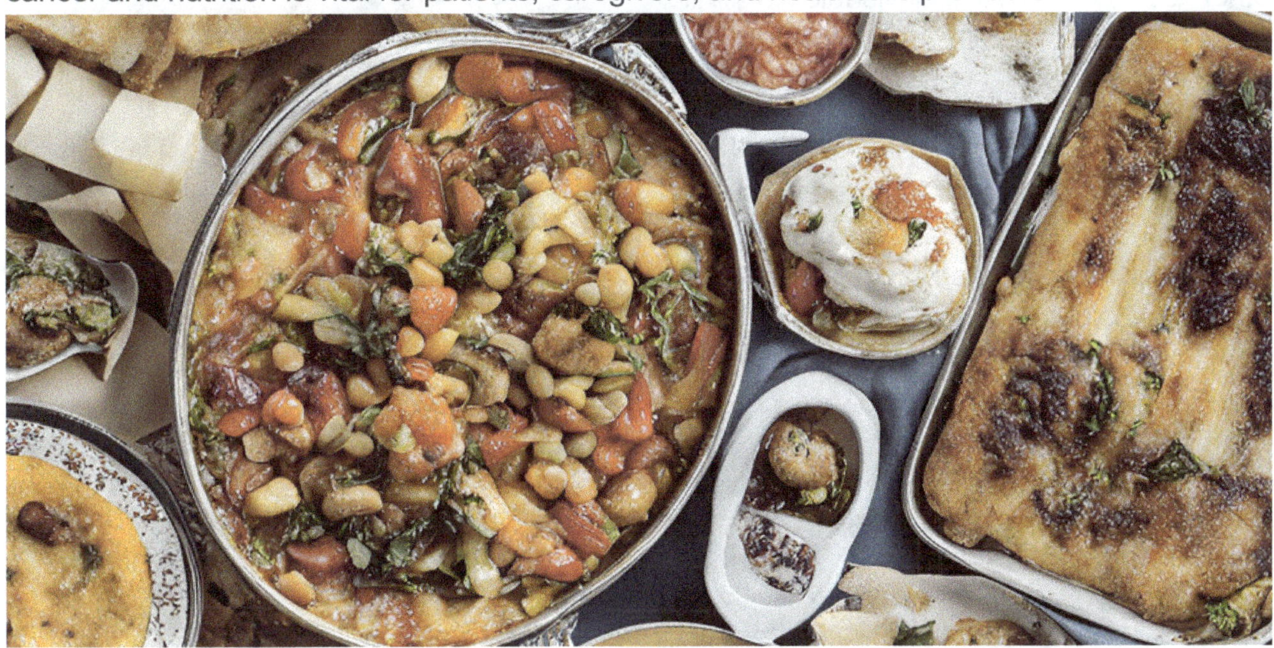

Nutrition plays a pivotal role in cancer prevention. Numerous studies have shown that diet and lifestyle choices can significantly influence the risk of developing cancer. A diet rich in fruits, vegetables, whole grains, and lean proteins is associated with a lower risk of several types of cancer.

Fruits and vegetables are packed with vitamins, minerals, antioxidants, and phytochemicals, which help protect cells from damage. Antioxidants like vitamin C, vitamin E, and beta-carotene neutralize harmful free radicals that can damage DNA and lead to cancer. Phytochemicals such as flavonoids, carotenoids, and polyphenols have been shown to have anti-cancer properties by inhibiting the growth of cancer cells and preventing the formation of new blood vessels that feed tumors.

Whole grains, such as brown rice, quinoa, and whole wheat, are excellent sources of fiber, which aids in digestion and helps maintain a healthy weight. Fiber also plays a role in regulating blood sugar levels and may reduce the risk of colorectal cancer.

Lean proteins, including fish, poultry, beans, and legumes, provide essential amino acids needed for tissue repair and immune function. Some studies suggest that a diet high in red and processed meats may increase the risk of colorectal and other cancers, so it's advisable to limit these and opt for healthier protein sources.

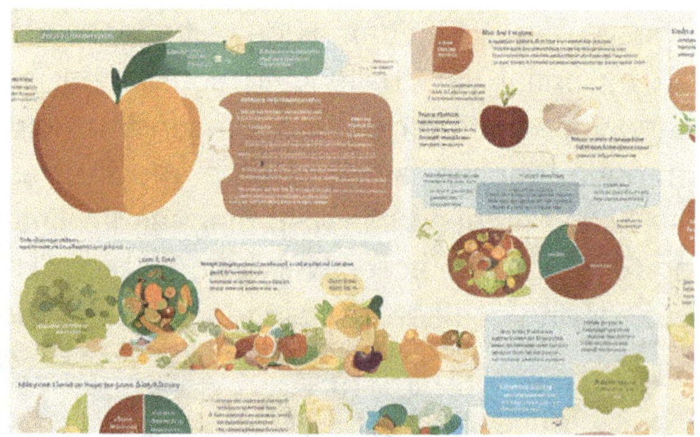

Maintaining a healthy weight through a balanced diet and regular physical activity is also crucial in cancer prevention. Obesity is a known risk factor for several cancers, including breast, colorectal, and endometrial cancers. Adopting a lifestyle that includes nutrient-rich foods, regular exercise, and avoiding tobacco and excessive alcohol consumption can significantly reduce the risk of developing cancer.

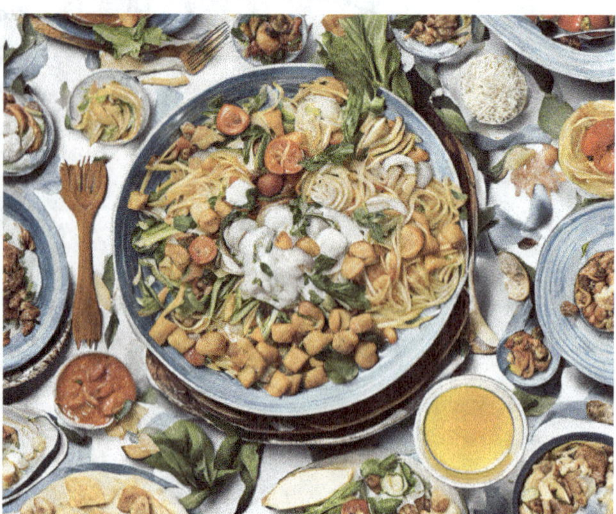

Cancer treatment often brings about a host of nutritional challenges. Chemotherapy, radiation therapy, and other treatments can cause side effects that impact a patient's ability to eat and digest food properly.

Here are some common nutritional challenges and ways to manage them:

- Nausea and Vomiting: These are common side effects of chemotherapy and radiation therapy. Eating small, frequent meals, and choosing bland, easy-to-digest foods like crackers, toast, and bananas can help. Ginger and peppermint tea may also alleviate nausea.
- Loss of Appetite: Treatment can reduce appetite, making it difficult to consume enough calories and nutrients. Eating small, nutrient-dense meals and snacks, and incorporating high-calorie, high-protein foods like nuts, cheese, and avocados can help.
- Taste Changes: Treatments can alter taste buds, making food taste metallic or bland. Enhancing flavors with herbs, spices, and marinades, and experimenting with different textures can make food more palatable.
- Mouth Sores and Difficulty Swallowing: Soft, moist foods like smoothies, soups, and mashed potatoes can be easier to eat. Avoiding acidic, spicy, or rough foods that can irritate the mouth is also important.
- Diarrhea and Constipation: These side effects can be managed by adjusting fiber intake. For diarrhea, eating low-fiber foods like white rice and bananas, and staying hydrated is crucial. For constipation, increasing fiber intake with fruits, vegetables, and whole grains, and drinking plenty of water can help.

Managing these nutritional challenges requires a flexible and individualized approach. Working with a dietitian or nutritionist can provide tailored advice and support to help patients maintain adequate nutrition during treatment.

Key Nutrients for Cancer Patients

- **Protein**: Essential for worn out or damaged tissues and immune function. Cancer patients often need more protein to rebuild muscle mass and support healing. Good sources include lean meats, eggs ,poultry, fish, dairy, beans, and legumes.

- **Carbohydrates**: Provide the primary source of energy. Whole grains, fruits, and vegetables are excellent sources that also provide fiber, vitamins, and minerals.

- **Fats**: Important for energy and cell function. Healthy fats from avocados, nuts, seeds, olive oil, and fatty fish like salmon provide essential fatty acids and help with nutrient absorption.

- **Vitamins and Minerals**: Vital for overall health and immune function. Vitamin C (found in citrus fruits, berries, and leafy greens) supports the immune system, while vitamin D (from sunlight, fortified foods, and fatty fish) is crucial for bone health. Iron (from red meat, beans, and spinach) is needed to prevent anemia, and calcium (from dairy, fortified plant milks, and leafy greens) supports bone strength.

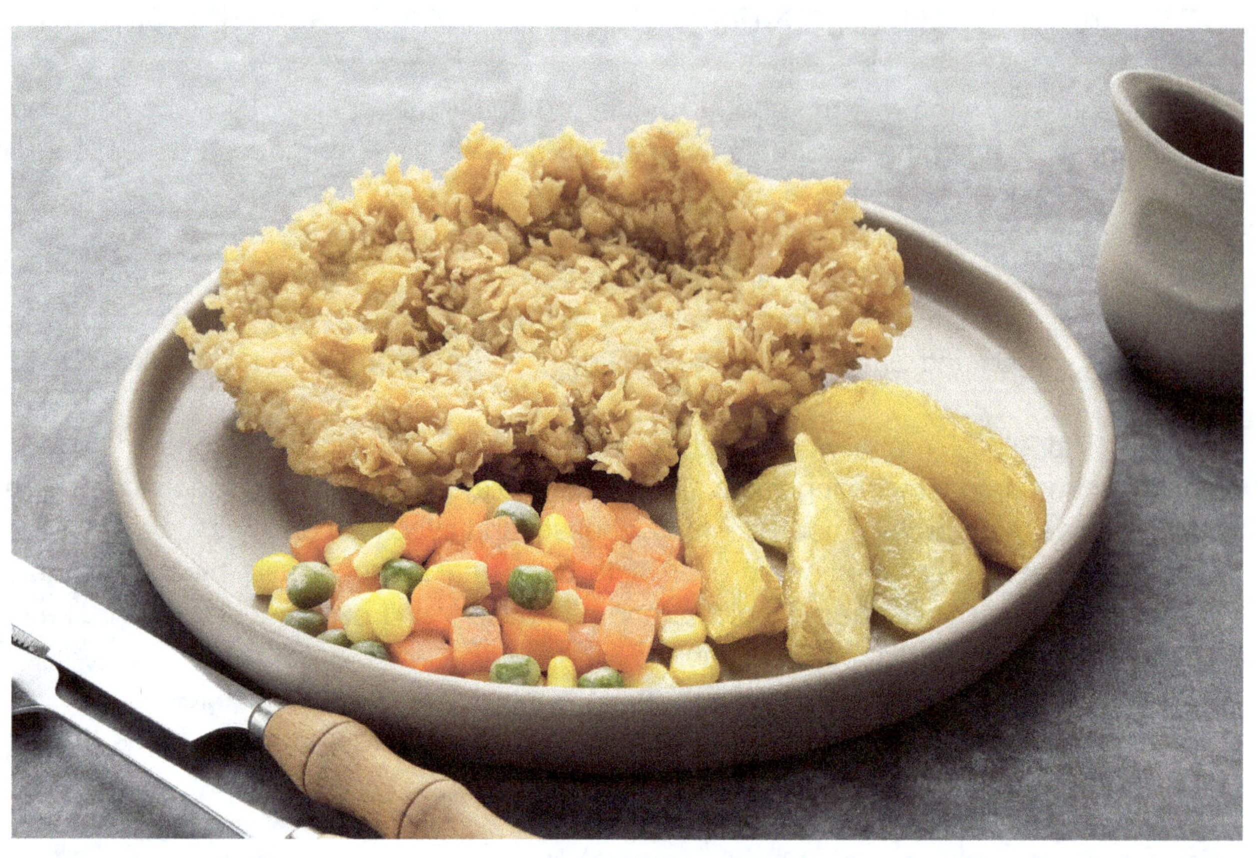

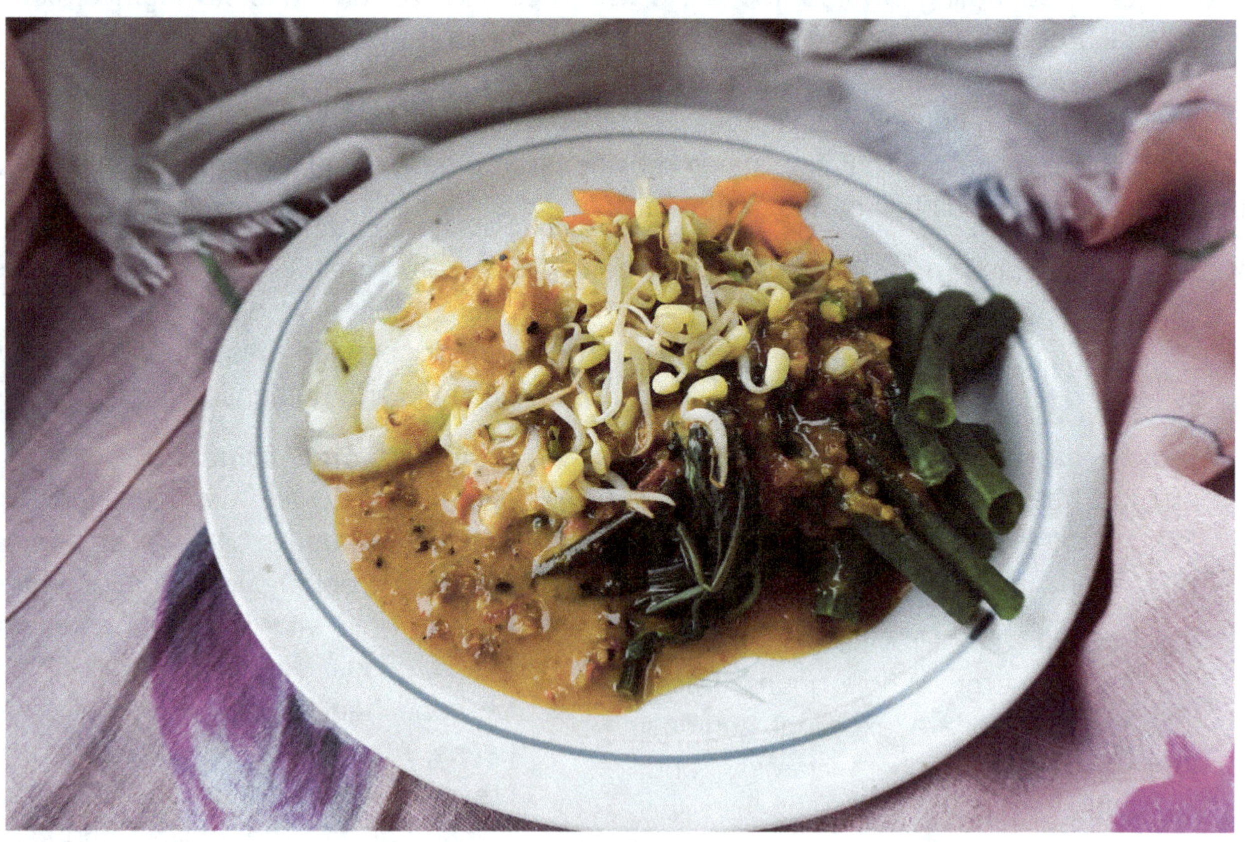

CHAPTER TWO

MANAGING SIDE EFFECTS THROUGH DIET

Cancer treatments such as chemotherapy, radiation, and surgery can cause various side effects that impact a patient's ability to eat and digest food. Managing these side effects through diet is essential for maintaining nutrition, improving comfort, and enhancing overall quality of life.

This chapter will explore common side effects and provide dietary strategies to help alleviate them.

NAUSEA AND VOMITING

Treatments for cancer frequently cause adverse effects like nausea and vomiting. The following advice can help you handle these symptoms:

- Eat Small, Frequent Meals: Large meals can be overwhelming, so aim for smaller, more frequent meals throughout the day.
- Choose Bland Foods: Foods like crackers, toast, plain rice, and bananas are easier on the stomach.
- Stay Hydrated: Sip on clear fluids like water, herbal teas, and broth throughout the day.
- Avoid Strong Smells: Strong odors can trigger nausea. Opt for cold or room-temperature foods to reduce smells.
- Try Ginger: Ginger has natural anti-nausea properties. Ginger tea, ginger ale, or ginger candies can be helpful.
- Rest After Eating: Sit up or recline slightly after meals to aid digestion and prevent nausea.

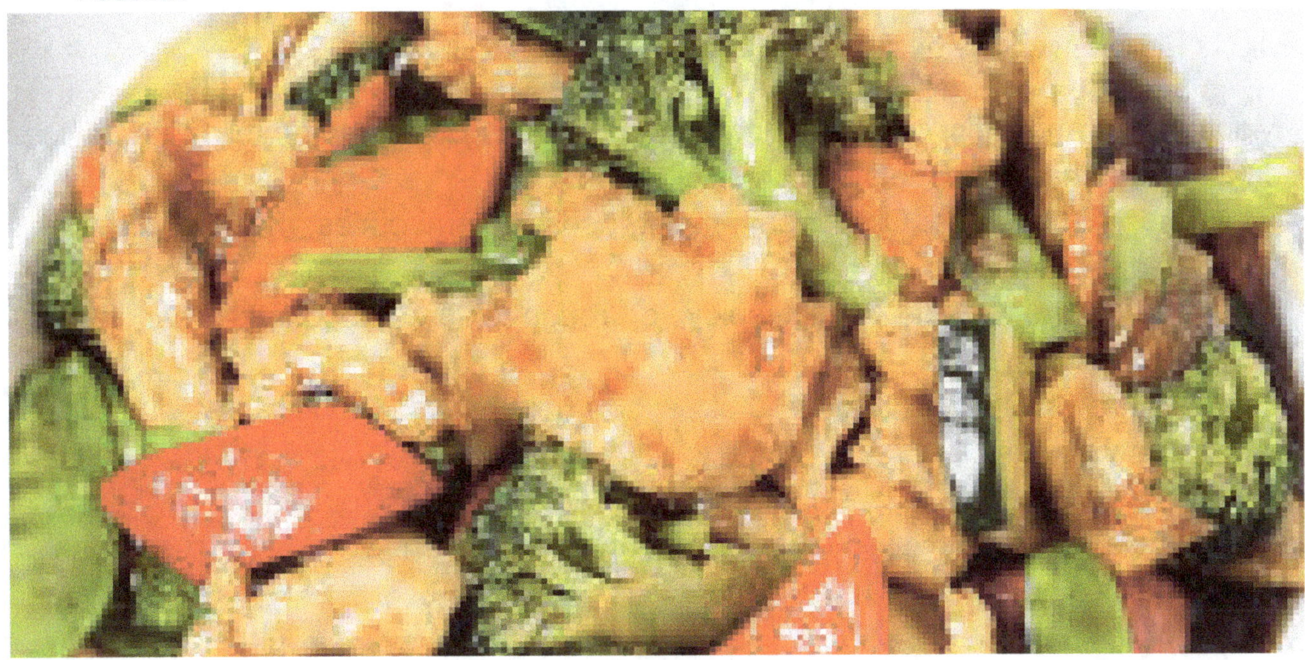

LOSS OF APPETITE

Loss of appetite can make it challenging to consume enough nutrients. Here are strategies to cope:
- Eat Small, Nutrient-Dense Meals: Focus on foods that are high in calories and nutrients, such as avocados, nuts, seeds, and nut butters.
- Enhance Flavors: Use herbs, spices, and marinades to make foods more appealing.
- Set a Schedule: Eat at regular times, even if you're not hungry, to establish a routine.
- Liquid Meals: Smoothies, shakes, and soups can be easier to consume and still provide essential nutrients.
- Keep Snacks Handy: Have easy-to-grab snacks available, such as trail mix, cheese, and yogurt.

TASTE CHANGES

Cancer treatments can alter taste, making food taste metallic, bland, or bitter. Here are ways to manage taste changes:
- Experiment with Flavors: Try adding citrus, herbs, and spices to enhance flavors.
- Use Plastic Utensils: If food tastes metallic, using plastic utensils instead of metal ones can help.
- Marinate Meats: Marinating meats can improve flavor and make them more palatable.
- Cold Foods: Cold or room-temperature foods might be more appealing if hot foods taste off.
- Rinse Your Mouth: Rinse your mouth with a baking soda and salt solution before eating to neutralize taste changes.

MOUTH SORES AND DIFFICULTY SWALLOWING

Mouth sores and difficulty swallowing can make eating painful. The following advice can help you handle these symptoms:
- Choose Soft Foods: Opt for soft, moist foods like smoothies, mashed potatoes, yogurt, and applesauce.
- Avoid Irritants: Avoid acidic, spicy, or rough-textured foods that can irritate mouth sores.
- Use Straws: Drinking through a straw can help bypass mouth sores and make swallowing easier.
- Stay Hydrated: Keep your mouth moist by sipping water frequently.
- Oral Care: Maintain good oral hygiene and use prescribed mouth rinses to help heal sores.

DIARRHEA

Diarrhea can lead to dehydration and nutrient loss. Here are dietary strategies to manage diarrhea:
- Increase Fluid Intake: Drink plenty of fluids like water, clear broths, and electrolyte-replenishing drinks.
- Eat Low-Fiber Foods: Choose foods that are low in fiber, such as white rice, bananas, applesauce, and white bread.
- Avoid Dairy: Some people with diarrhea may be sensitive to lactose, so it might be helpful to avoid dairy products.

CONSTIPATION

Constipation is another common side effect of cancer treatments. Here are ways to alleviate constipation through diet:
- Increase Fiber Intake: Foods high in fiber, such as whole grains, fruits, vegetables, and legumes, can help regulate bowel movements.
- Stay Hydrated: Drink plenty of water to help fiber work effectively.
- Exercise: Regular physical activity can help stimulate digestion and relieve constipation.
- Prunes and Prune Juice: Prunes and prune juice have natural laxative properties that can help relieve constipation.
- Avoid Processed Foods: Limit intake of processed and low-fiber foods, which can contribute to constipation.

FATIGUE

Fatigue is a common issue for cancer patients, affecting their energy levels and overall well-being. Here are dietary strategies to combat fatigue:
- Eat Balanced Meals: Ensure your meals include a balance of protein, carbohydrates, and healthy fats to provide sustained energy.
- Stay Hydrated: Dehydration can contribute to fatigue, so drink plenty of fluids throughout the day.
- Limit Caffeine and Sugar: While caffeine and sugary foods can provide a temporary energy boost, they can also lead to energy crashes. Opt for complex
- carbohydrates and protein-rich snacks instead.
- Plan Meals Around Energy Levels: Prepare meals and snacks when you have the most energy, and keep easy-to-eat options available for when you feel tired.
- Consider Nutritional Supplements: If you're struggling to meet your nutritional needs through food alone, consult with your healthcare team about the potential benefits
- of nutritional supplements.

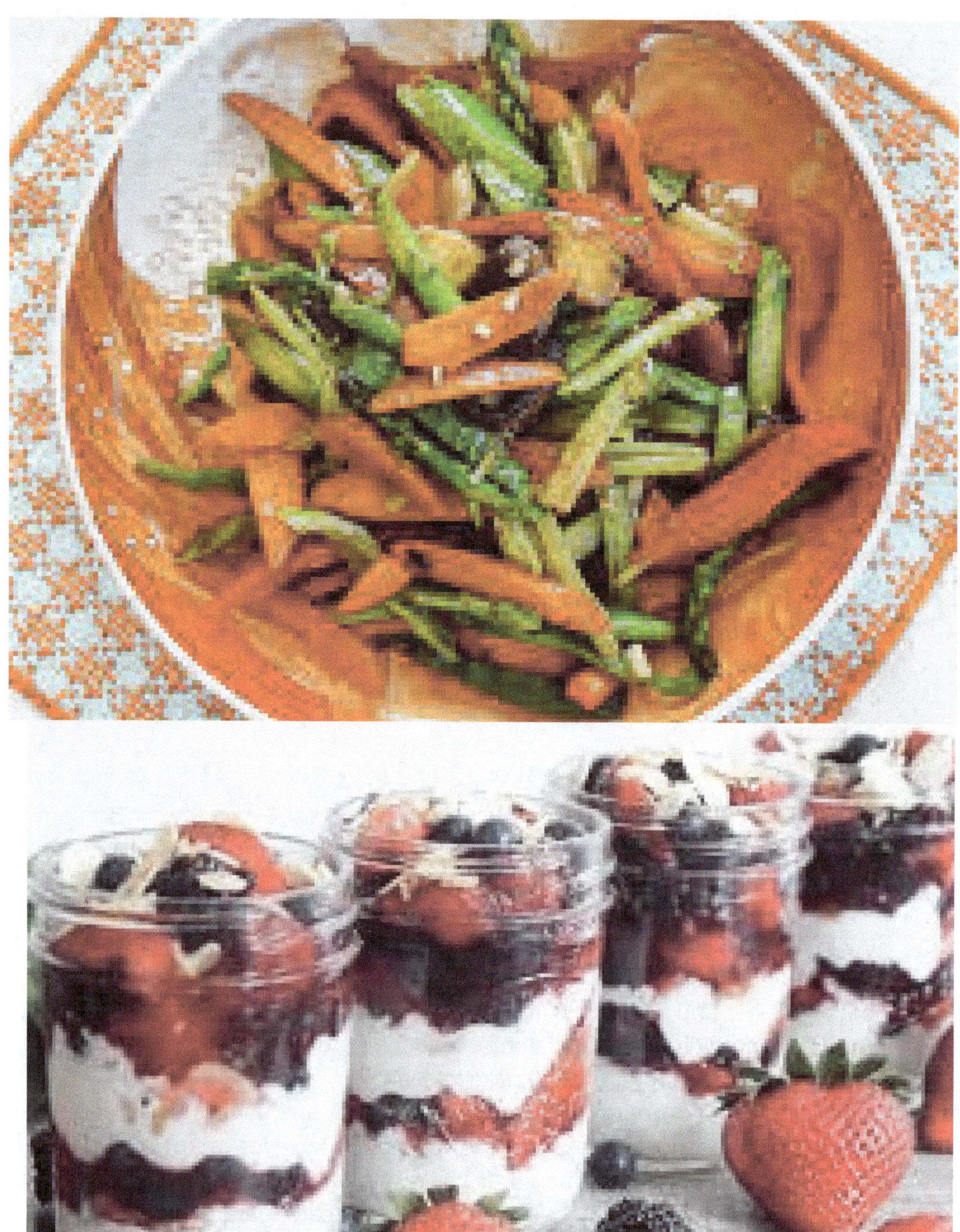

CHAPTER THREE

Meal Planning Strategies for Cancer Patients

Effective meal planning is crucial for cancer patients, as it helps ensure that they receive the necessary nutrients to support their health and manage the side effects of treatment. Proper meal planning can improve energy levels, maintain a healthy weight, and enhance overall well-being. This chapter will guide you through creating personalized meal plans tailored to your specific needs and preferences.

UNDERSTANDING NUTRITIONAL NEEDS

Macronutrients, which include carbohydrates, proteins, and fats, provide the energy and building blocks necessary for bodily functions. Micronutrients, such as vitamins and minerals, play critical roles in supporting metabolic processes and maintaining health.

Some cancer treatments may require specific dietary adjustments. For example, a low-fiber diet may be necessary for patients experiencing gastrointestinal issues, while a soft diet can be helpful for those with swallowing difficulties.

ROLE OF PROTEIN IN CANCER CARE

Protein is a cornerstone of nutrition for cancer patients, supporting healing, muscle maintenance, and immune function. By understanding the importance of protein and incorporating a variety of protein-rich foods into your diet, you can enhance your nutritional status and overall well-being during treatment.

Functions of Protein

- Tissue Repair and Growth: Proteins are essential for repairing and regenerating tissues. This is particularly important for cancer patients who may experience tissue damage from treatments like surgery, chemotherapy, or radiation.

- Muscle Maintenance: Adequate protein intake helps maintain muscle mass, which can be compromised during cancer treatment due to reduced physical activity and side effects such as fatigue and appetite loss.

- Immune Function: Proteins are crucial for the production of antibodies and immune system cells. A strong immune system is essential for fighting infections and supporting overall health.

- Enzyme and Hormone Production: Proteins are involved in the creation of enzymes and hormones that regulate various bodily functions, including metabolism and the healing process.

ROLES OF CARBOHYDRATES IN CANCER CARE

Carbohydrates are a fundamental source of energy, providing the fuel needed for daily activities and bodily functions. By understanding the importance of carbohydrates and incorporating a variety of carbohydrate-rich foods into your diet, you can enhance your energy levels, support overall health, and manage treatment-related side effects.

Functions of Carbohydrates

- Energy Production: Carbohydrates are the body's primary source of energy. They are broken down into glucose, which is used by cells to perform essential functions. This is especially important for cancer patients who may experience fatigue and require adequate energy to sustain their activities and treatment regimen.

- Digestive Health: Carbohydrates, particularly those high in fiber, support digestive health. Fiber aids in maintaining regular bowel movements, which can be disrupted by cancer treatments such as chemotherapy. It also helps in preventing constipation, a common side effect of many cancer treatments.

- Immune Support: Certain carbohydrates, such as those found in fruits, vegetables, and whole grains, are rich in vitamins, minerals, and antioxidants that support the immune system. A strong immune system is crucial for cancer patients to combat infections and aid in the recovery process.

- Blood Sugar Regulation: Complex carbohydrates, which are slowly digested, help maintain stable blood sugar levels. This is important for cancer patients who need consistent energy levels throughout the day and to avoid energy spikes and crashes.

- Protein-Sparing Effect: Adequate carbohydrate intake ensures that proteins are used for their primary roles, such as tissue repair and immune function, rather than being used for energy. This is vital for maintaining muscle mass and overall health during cancer treatment.

ROLE OF FATS IN CANCER CARE

Fats are a vital component of nutrition, providing essential fatty acids, supporting cell function, and aiding in the absorption of fat-soluble vitamins.

Functions of Fats

- Absorption of Vitamins: Fats aid in the absorption of fat-soluble vitamins (A, D, E, and K). These vitamins are important for immune function, bone health, antioxidant protection, and blood clotting.

- Energy Source: Fats are a concentrated source of energy, providing more than twice the calories per gram compared to carbohydrates and proteins. This is especially important for cancer patients who may have higher energy needs or difficulty maintaining weight due to treatment side effects.

- Cell Function and Structure: Fats are crucial for building and maintaining cell membranes. They play a key role in cell signaling, which is essential for immune function and overall cellular health.

- Anti-Inflammatory Properties: Certain types of fats, such as omega-3 fatty acids found in fish, flaxseeds, and walnuts, have anti-inflammatory properties. These can help reduce inflammation in the body, which is beneficial for cancer patients experiencing inflammation due to the disease or its treatment.

- Hormone Production: Fats are involved in the production of hormones that regulate various bodily functions, including metabolism, immune response, and reproductive health.

ROLE OF VITAMINA & MINERALS IN CANCER CARE

Vitamins and minerals are cornerstones of nutrition for cancer patients, supporting immune function, antioxidant protection, bone health, red blood cell production, energy metabolism, wound healing, and nervous system function.

Functions of Vitamins & Minerals

- Immune Support: Vitamins and minerals such as vitamin C, vitamin D, zinc, and selenium are crucial for maintaining a strong immune system. A robust immune system helps cancer patients fight off infections and supports overall health.

- Antioxidant Protection: Vitamins like vitamin C, vitamin E, and beta-carotene (a form of vitamin A) act as antioxidants. They protect cells from damage caused by free radicals, which can be particularly beneficial for cancer patients as oxidative stress is often elevated during treatment.

- Bone Health: Calcium and vitamin D are essential for maintaining strong bones. Cancer patients, especially those undergoing certain treatments like hormone therapy, may be at increased risk for bone density loss, making these nutrients vital for bone health.

- Red Blood Cell Production: Iron, vitamin B12, and folate are essential for the production of red blood cells. Adequate levels of these nutrients help prevent anemia, which can cause fatigue and weakness in cancer patients.

CREATING A BALANCED MEAL PLAN

1. Assess Your Needs

- Consult with your healthcare team, including a dietitian, to understand your specific nutritional requirements and any dietary restrictions.
- Consider factors such as treatment stage, side effects, and personal preferences.

2. Plan Your Meals

- Breakfast: Aim for a protein-rich breakfast to start your day with energy. Examples include Greek yogurt with berries, oatmeal with nuts, or a vegetable omelet.
- Lunch: Incorporate lean proteins, whole grains, and vegetables. A quinoa salad with chicken, mixed greens, and avocado is a good option.
- Dinner: Focus on a balanced meal with protein, whole grains, and vegetables. Try grilled salmon with brown rice and steamed broccoli.
- Snacks: Include nutrient-dense snacks to keep your energy levels up. Options include nuts, fruit, cheese, or hummus with vegetables.

3. Batch Cooking and Freezing

- Prepare large batches of meals and freeze them in individual portions. This saves time and ensures you always have a nutritious meal ready.
- Soups, stews, casseroles, and grain-based salads are great for batch cooking.

4. Incorporate Variety

- Rotate different foods and recipes to ensure a wide range of nutrients and prevent meal fatigue.
- Experiment with new recipes and ingredients to keep meals interesting and enjoyable.

5. Adapting to Treatment Side Effects

- Modify meal plans based on how you feel each day. For example, if you're experiencing nausea, opt for bland, easy-to-digest foods.
- Keep a variety of foods on hand so you can adjust your meals according to your appetite and preferences.

6. Stay Flexible

- Listen to your body and adjust your meal plans as needed. It's important to stay flexible and make changes based on how you're feeling.
- Don't be afraid to seek help from family, friends, or caregivers in preparing meals.

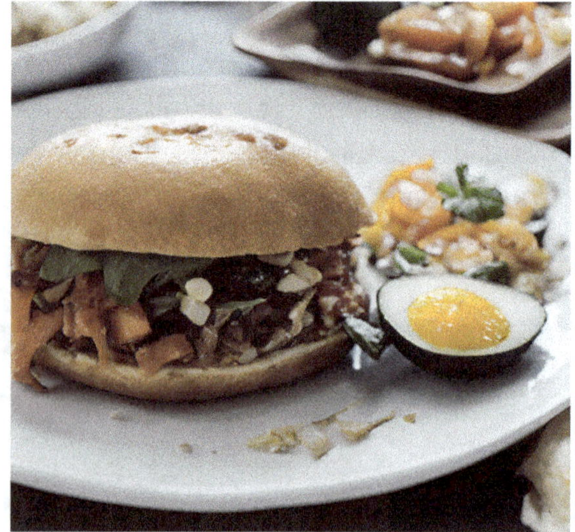

TIPS FOR SUCCESSFUL MEAL PLANNING

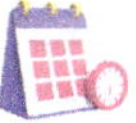 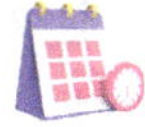  

- Keep a Food Diary: Track what you eat and how you feel. This helps to identify patterns and adjust diet accordingly.
- Grocery Shopping Tips: Make a shopping list based on your meal plan to ensure you have all the necessary ingredients. Focus on whole, minimally processed foods.
- Stay Organized: Use containers to portion out meals and snacks for the week. Ensure to label them with dates to constantly keep track of freshness.
- Hydration: Always include hydrating beverages and water-rich foods in your meal plan.

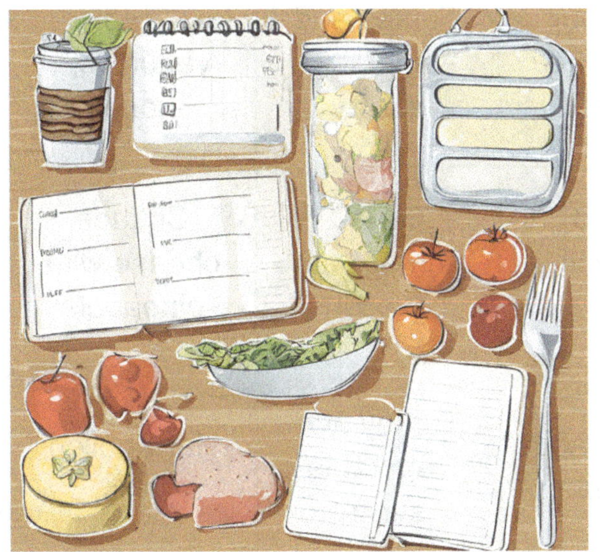 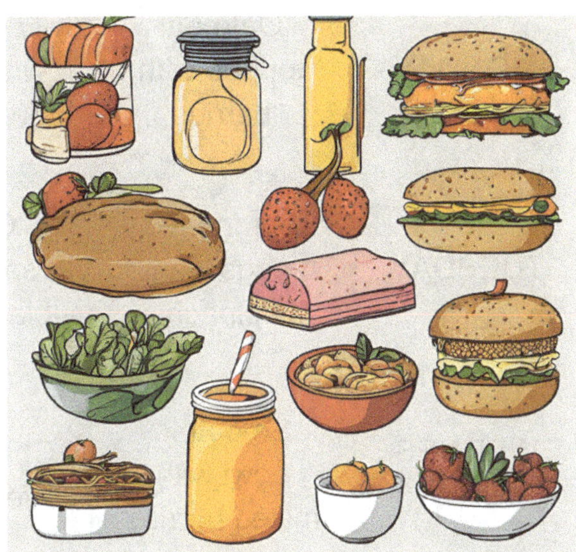

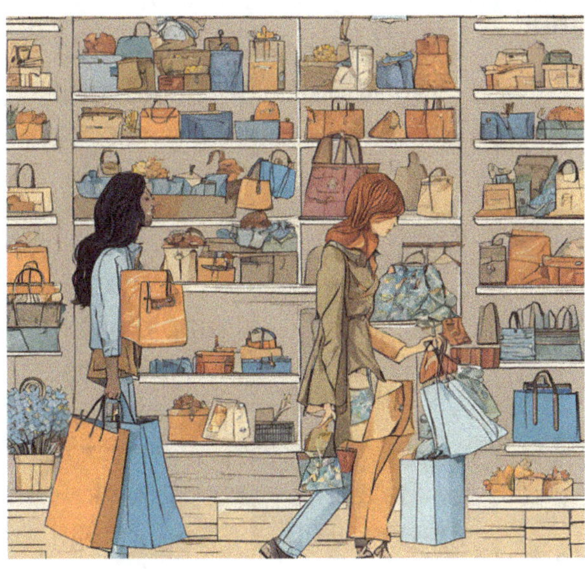 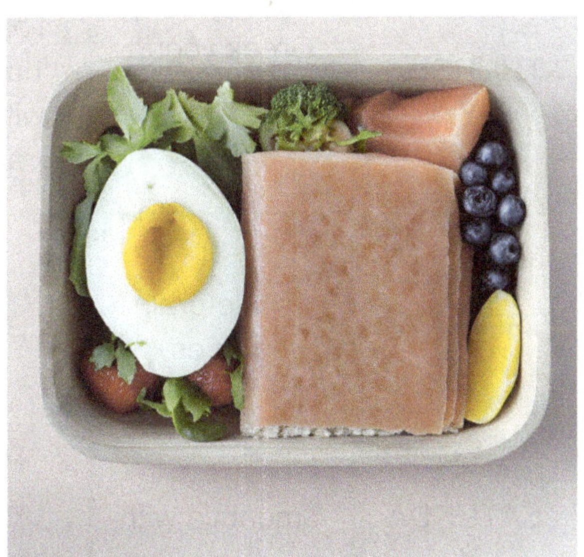

A 7 DAY MEAL PLAN GUIDE

DAY	BREAKFAST	LAUNCH	DINNER	SNACKS
SUNDAY	Smoothie with spinach	Grilled chicken salads	Baked salmon with quinoa	Hummus with carrot sticks.
MONDAY	Oatmeal topped with berries	Lentil soup with whole-grain bread	Turkey and vegetable stir-fry	Greek yogurt with honey
TUESDAY	Scrambled eggs with spinach	Quinoa salad with black beans	Grilled shrimp with couscous	Cottage cheese with pineapple
WEDNES DAY	Smoothie bowl with mixed berries	Chicken and vegetable	Turkey and vegetable stir-fry	Hard-boiled eggs.
THURSDA Y	Greek yogurt with sliced banana	Tomato and basil pasta with whole-grain penne.	Beef and vegetable stew	Fresh fruit salad, trail mix.
FRIDAY	Whole-grain waffles	Spinach	Grilled tofu with stir-fried vegetables	Edamame, apple slices with cheese
SATURDA Y	Smoothie with kale	Roasted vegetable	Baked chicken with brown rice	Greek yogurt with granola.

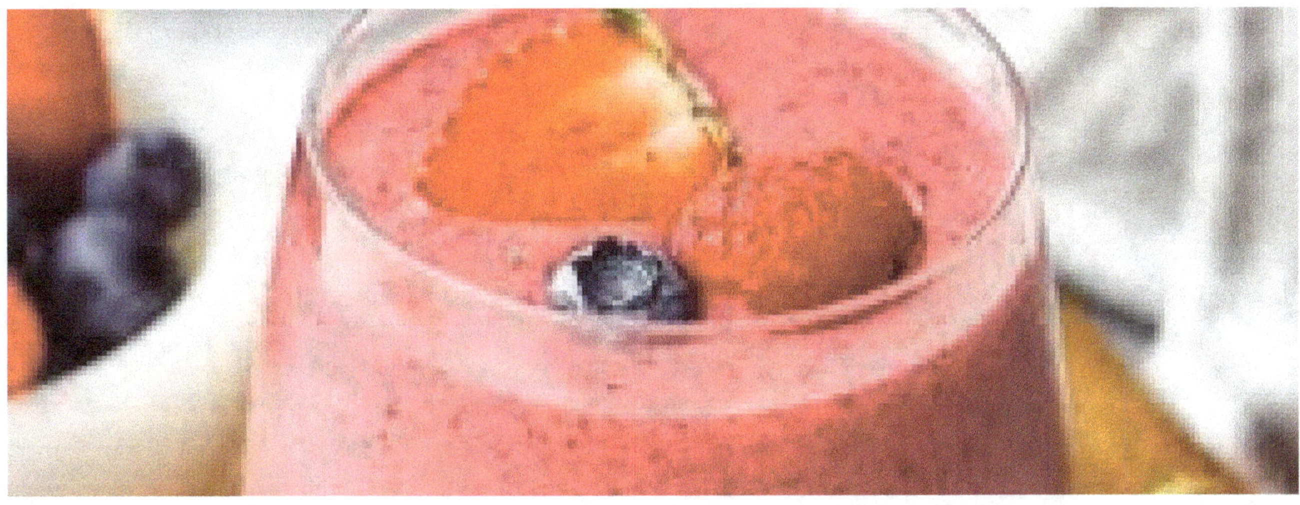

 Prep time
5 minutes

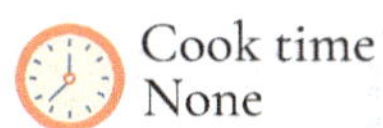 Cook time
None

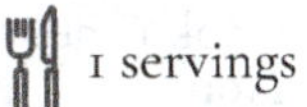 1 servings

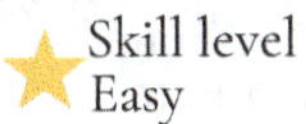 Skill level
Easy

Berry Smoothie

INGREDIENTS

BREAKFAST

1 cup mixed berries

1 banana

1 cup spinach

1 cup almond milk

INSTRUCTIONS

1. Add All ingredients in a blender.
2. Blend until smooth.
3. Pour into a tumbler or glass and serve right away.

NUTRITIONAL FACTS

Calories: 150

Protein: 3g

Carbohydrates: 35g

Fat: 2g

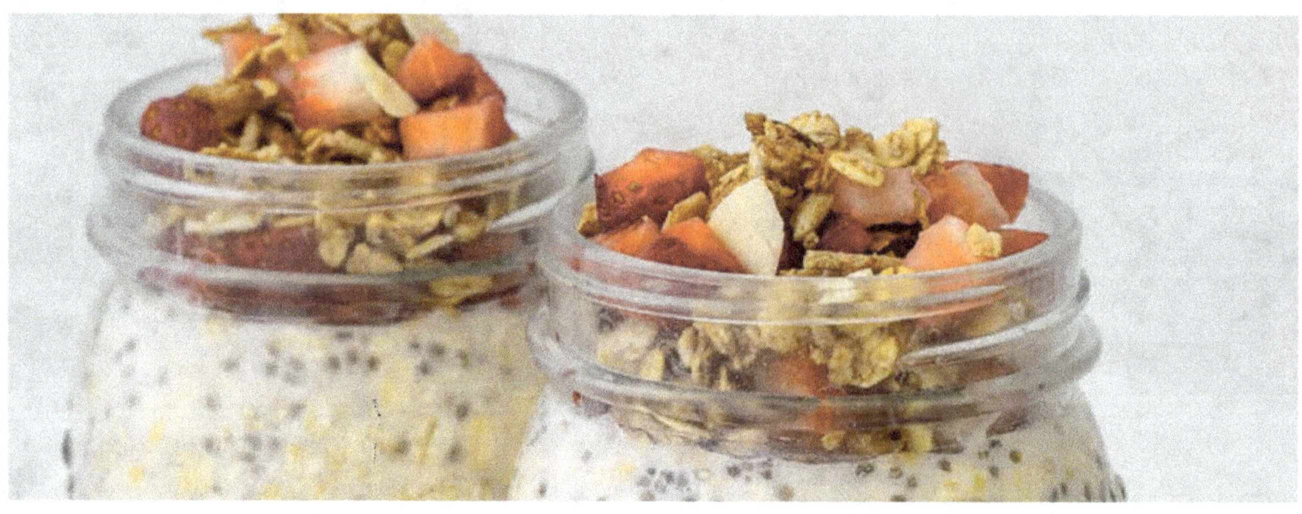

 **Prep time**
5 minutes

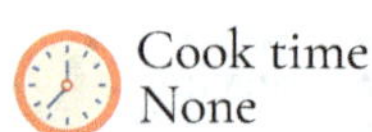 **Cook time**
None

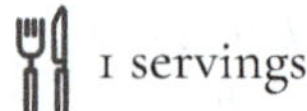 1 servings

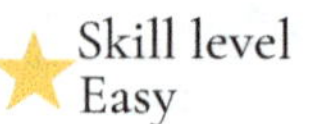 **Skill level**
Easy

Overnight Oats

INGREDIENTS

BREAKFAST

1/2 cup rolled oats

1/2 cup almond milk

1 tablespoon chia seeds

1 tablespoon honey

1/4 cup mixed berries

NUTRITIONAL FACTS

Calories: 250

Protein: 6g

Carbohydrates: 45g

Fat: 5g

INSTRUCTIONS

1. In a jar, combine oats, almond milk, chia seeds, and honey.
2. Stir and shake very well, cover the jar, and allow to refrigerate overnight.
3. In the morning, top with mixed berries and serve.

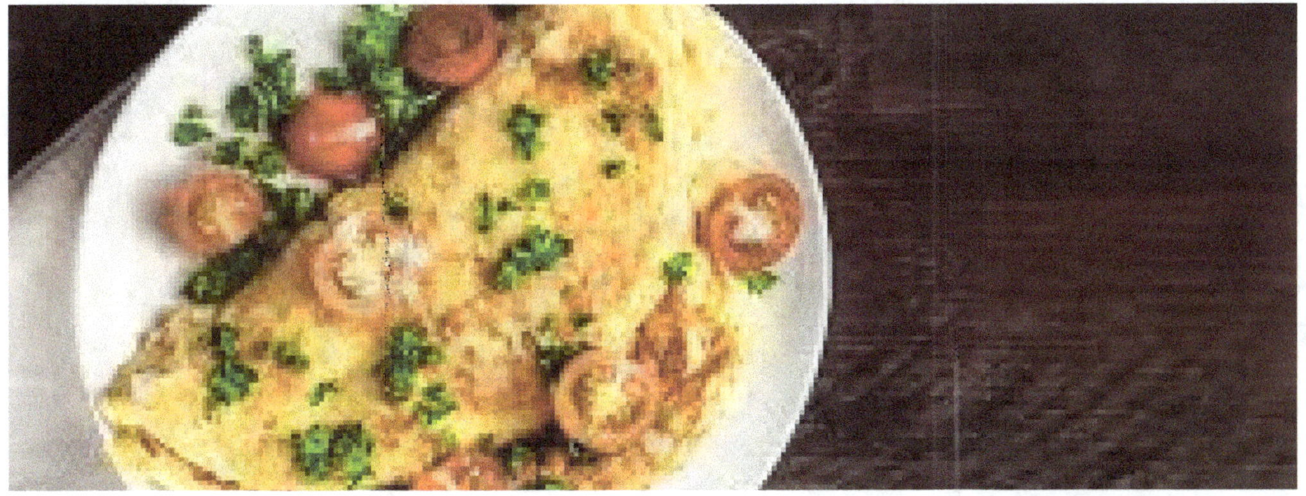

Prep time
5 minutes

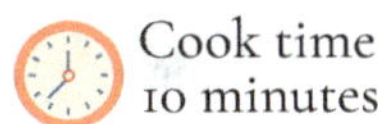
Cook time
10 minutes

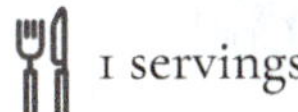
1 servings

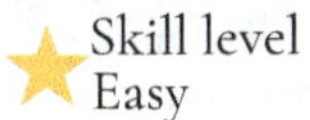
Skill level
Easy

Veggie Omelette

INGREDIENTS

2 eggs

1/4 cup diced bell peppers

1/4 cup chopped spinach

1/4 cup diced tomatoes

1 tablespoon olive oil

Salt and pepper to taste

NUTRITIONAL FACTS

Calories: 200

Protein: 12g

Carbohydrates: 6g

Fat: 15g

INSTRUCTIONS

1. Beat the eggs in a bowl and add salt and pepper to season.
2. Apply medium heat to warm the olive oil in a non-stick pan.
3. Add bell peppers, spinach, and tomatoes to the pan and cook until softened.
4. Pour the beaten eggs over the vegetables and allow to cook until set.
5. Fold the omelette in half and serve.

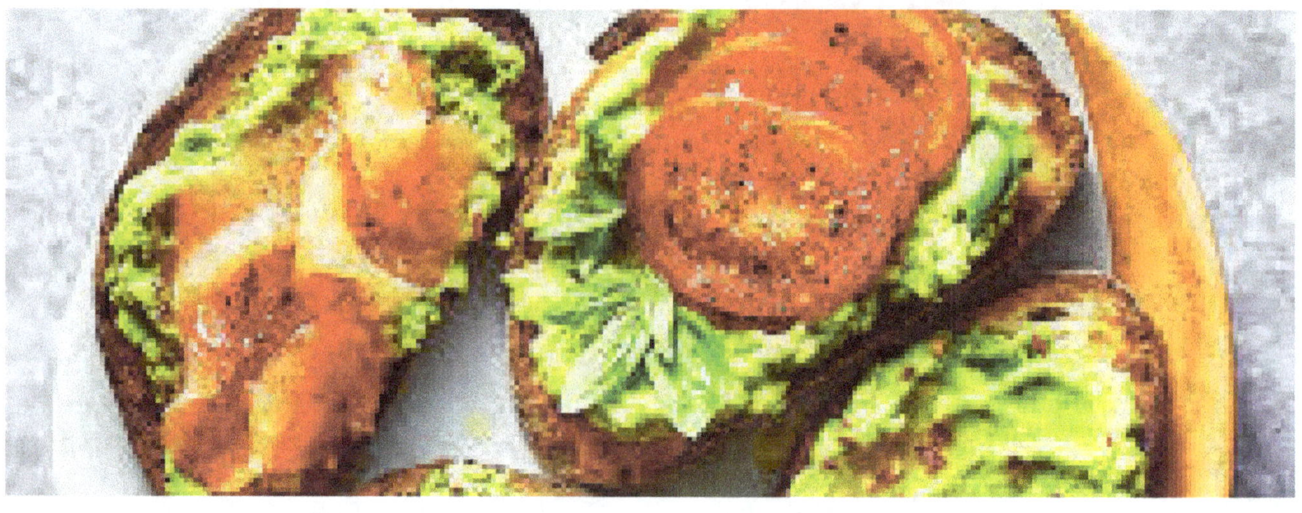

Prep time
5 minutes

Cook time
5 minutes

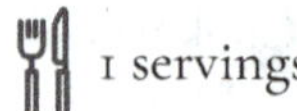
1 servings

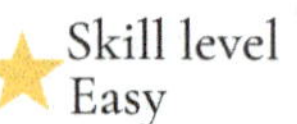
Skill level
Easy

Avocado Toast

BREAKFAST

INGREDIENTS

1 ripe avocado

2 slices whole grain bread

1 tablespoon olive oil

Salt and pepper to taste

Optional toppings: cherry tomatoes, red pepper flakes, poached egg

NUTRITIONAL FACTS

Calories: 300

Protein: 6g

Carbohydrates: 35g

Fat: 18g

INSTRUCTIONS

1. Toast the bread slices.
2. Mash the ripe avocado in a bowl and season with salt and pepper.
3. Spread the mashed avocado on the toasted bread.
4. Drizzle with olive oil and add optional toppings as desired.

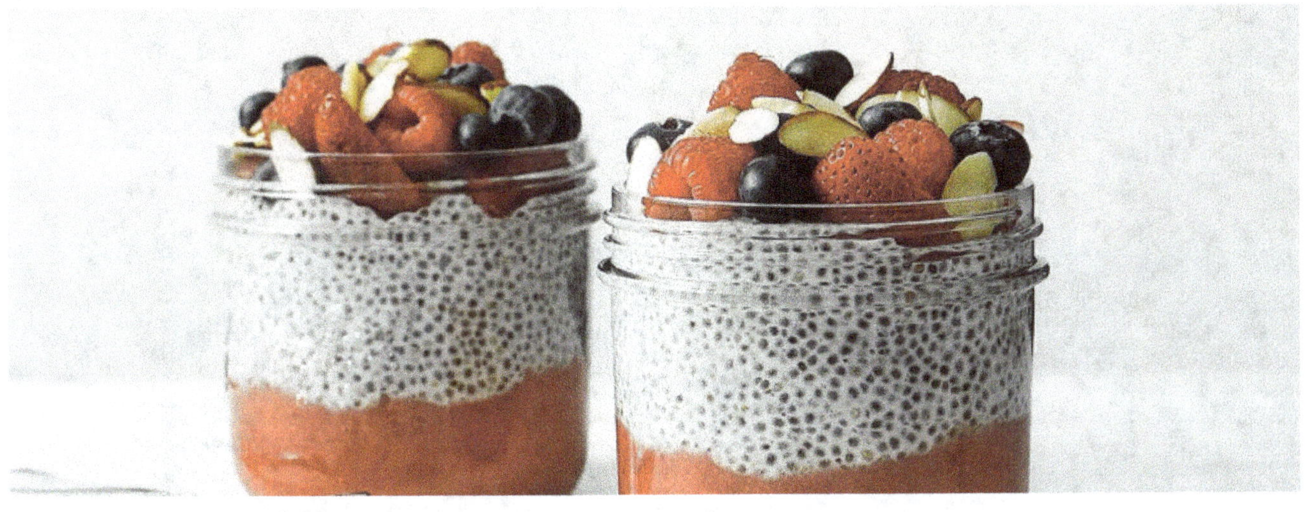

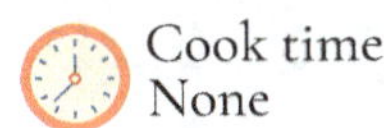

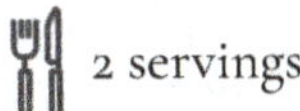

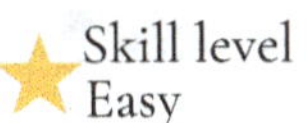

Chia Seed Pudding

BREAKFAST

INGREDIENTS

1/4 cup chia seeds

1 cup almond milk

1 tablespoon honey

1/2 teaspoon vanilla extract

Fresh fruit for topping

NUTRITIONAL FACTS

Calories: 150

Protein: 4g

Carbohydrates: 20g

Fat: 7g

INSTRUCTIONS

1. In a bowl, combine chia seeds, almond milk, honey, and vanilla extract.
2. Stir well and refrigerate for at least 2 hours or overnight until thickened.
3. Top with fresh fruit before serving.

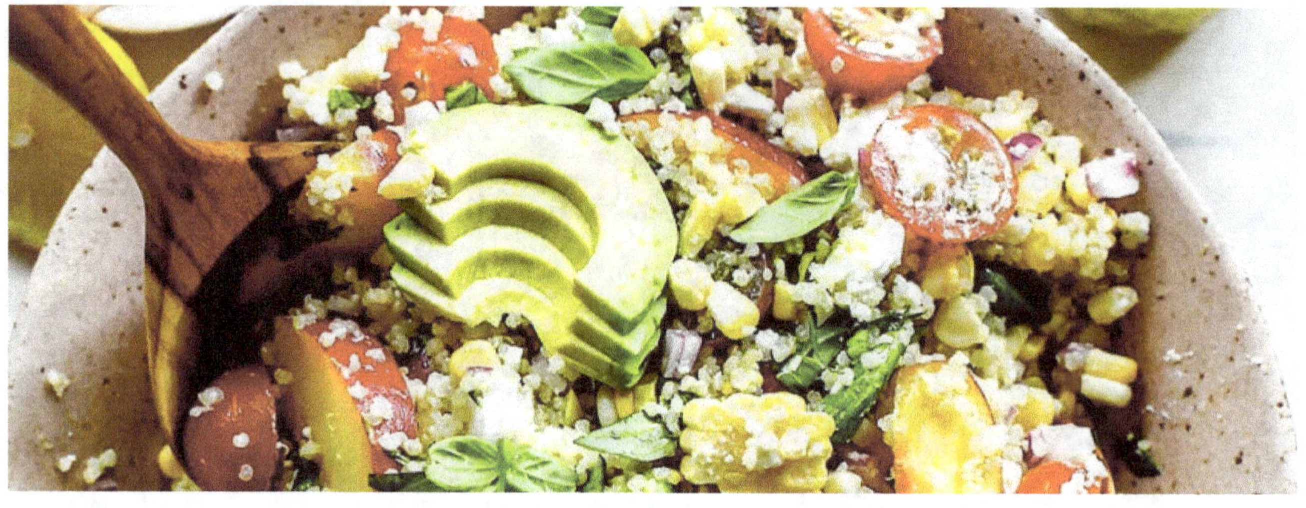

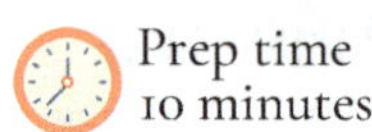 **Prep time**
10 minutes

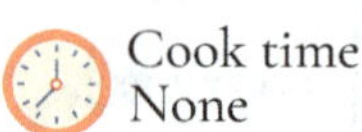 **Cook time**
None

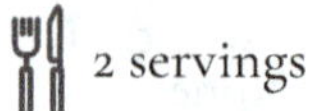 2 servings

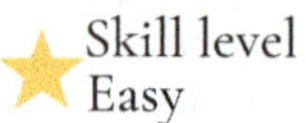 **Skill level**
Easy

Quinoa Salad

LUNCH

INGREDIENTS

1 cup cooked quinoa

1/2 cup chopped cucumber

1/2 cup cherry tomatoes, halved

1/4 cup chopped red onion

1/4 cup chopped parsley

2 tablespoons olive oil

1 tablespoon lemon juice

Salt and pepper to taste

NUTRITIONAL FACTS

Calories: 200

Protein: 5g

Carbohydrates: 28g

Fat: 8g

INSTRUCTIONS

1. In a large bowl, combine quinoa, cucumber, cherry tomatoes, red onion, and parsley.
2. In a small bowl, whisk together the olive oil, lemon juice, salt, and pepper.
3. Pour the dressing over the salad, then toss to combine.

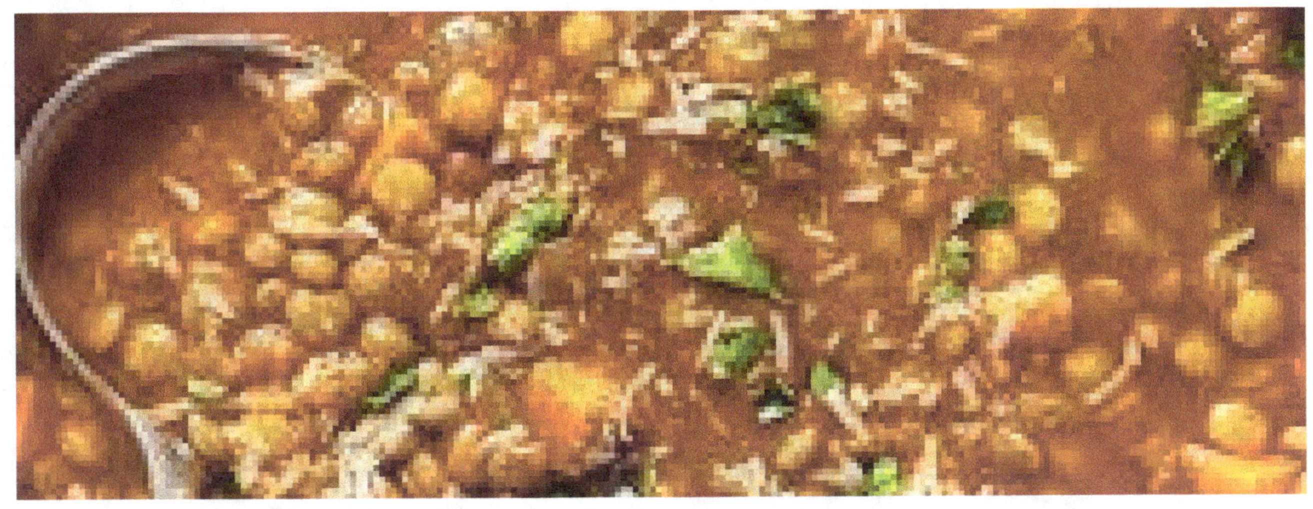

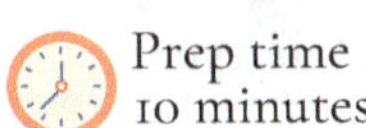 Prep time
10 minutes

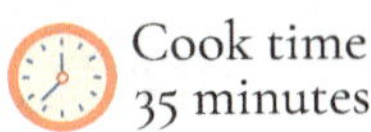 Cook time
35 minutes

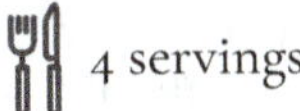 4 servings

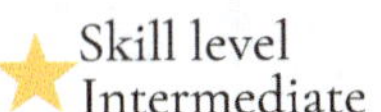 Skill level
Intermediate

Lentil Soup

INGREDIENTS

1 cup lentils, rinsed

1 carrot, diced *1 onion, chopped

1 celery stalk, diced

2 cloves garlic, minced

4cups vegetable broth

1 can (14 oz) diced tomatoes

1 teaspoon cumin

1 teaspoon paprika

2 tablespoons olive oil

- Salt and pepper to taste

NUTRITIONAL FACTS

Calories: 250

Protein: 12g

Carbohydrates: 40g

Fat: 8g

INSTRUCTIONS

1. In a large pot, heat the olive oil over medium heat. Add onion, carrot, and celery, and cook until softened.

2. Add garlic, cumin, and paprika, and cook for 1 minute.

3. Add lentils, vegetable broth, and diced tomatoes. Bring to a boil.

4. Reduce heat and simmer for 30-35 minutes, until lentils are tender.

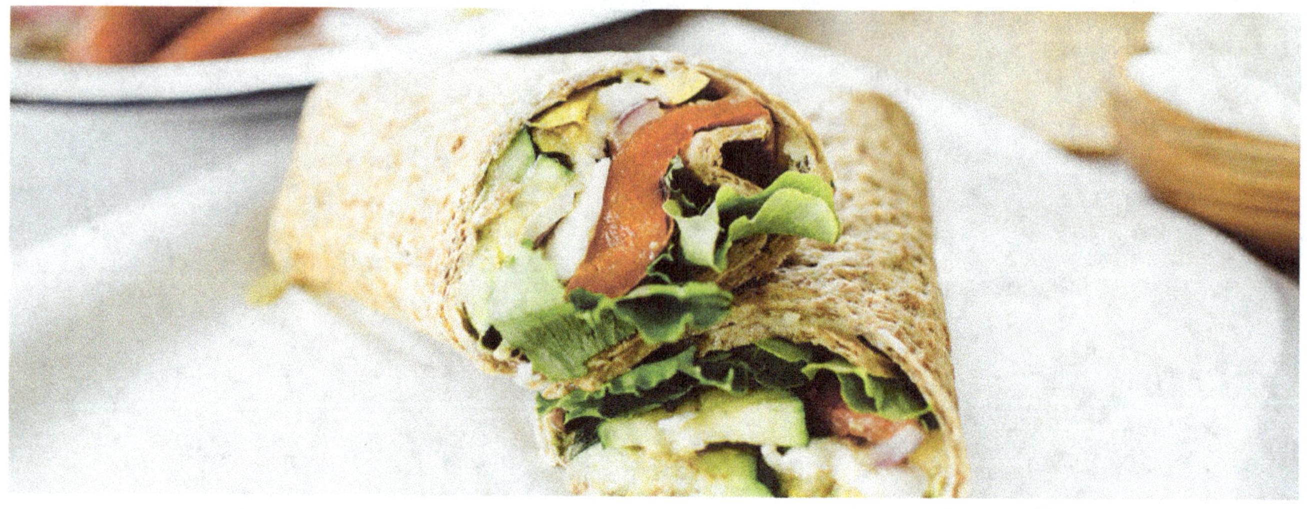

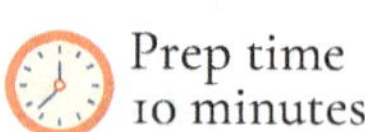 Prep time
10 minutes

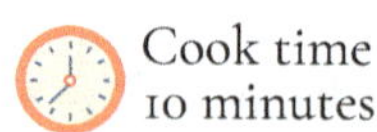 Cook time
10 minutes

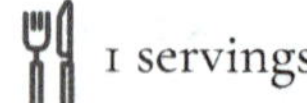 1 servings

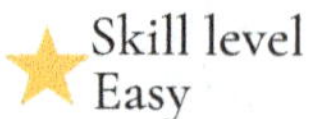 Skill level
Easy

Grilled veggie wrap

INGREDIENTS

1 large tortilla wrap

1/2 cup grilled zucchini slices

1/2 cup grilled bell pepper slices

1/4 cup hummus

1/4 cup fresh spinach leaves

2 tablespoons feta cheese, crumbled

NUTRITIONAL FACTS

Calories: 250

Protein: 10g

Carbohydrates: 35g

Fat: 10g

INSTRUCTIONS

1. Spread hummus evenly over the tortilla wrap.
2. Layer grilled zucchini, bell pepper slices, spinach leaves, and feta cheese.
3. Roll up the tortilla tightly and slice in half.

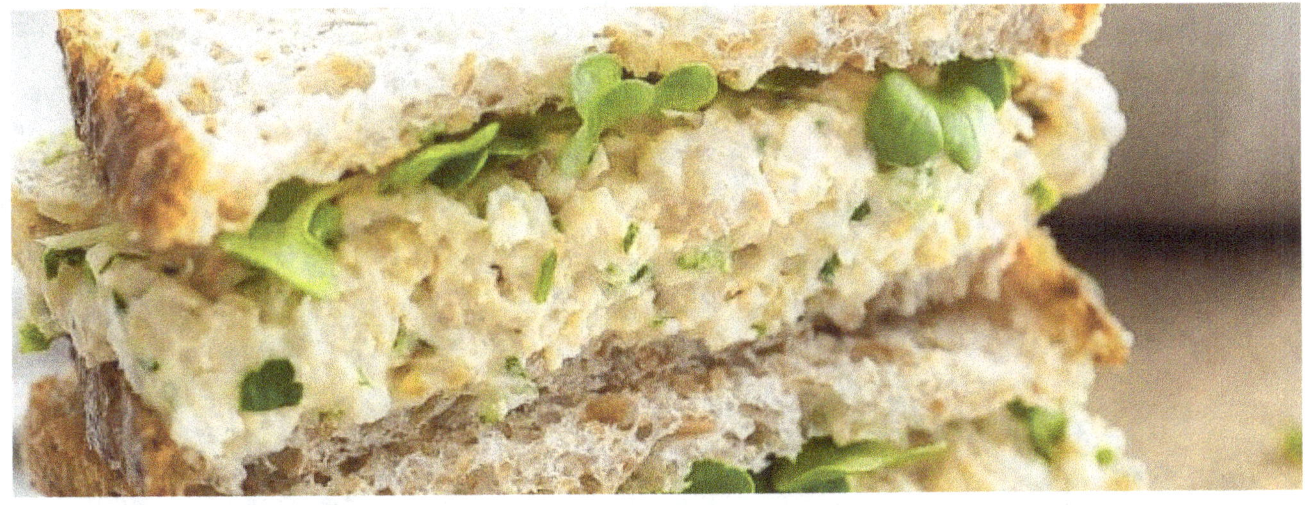

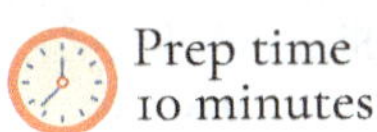 Prep time
10 minutes

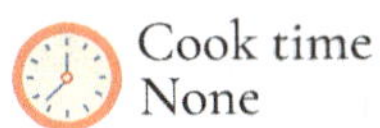 Cook time
None

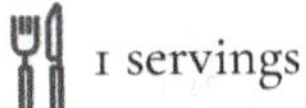 1 servings

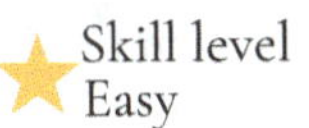 Skill level
Easy

Chickpea salad sandwich

INGREDIENTS

1 can (15 oz) chickpeas, drained and rinsed

1/4 cup diced celery

1/4 cup diced red onion

2 tablespoons vegan mayonnaise

1 tablespoon lemon juice

Salt and pepper to taste

NUTRITIONAL FACTS

Calories: 300

Protein: 12g

Carbohydrates: 45g

Fat: 8g

INSTRUCTIONS

1. In a bowl, mash chickpeas with a fork until slightly chunky.
2. Stir in celery, red onion, vegan mayonnaise, lemon juice, salt, and pepper.
3. Spread the chickpea mixture onto one slice of bread and top with the other slice.

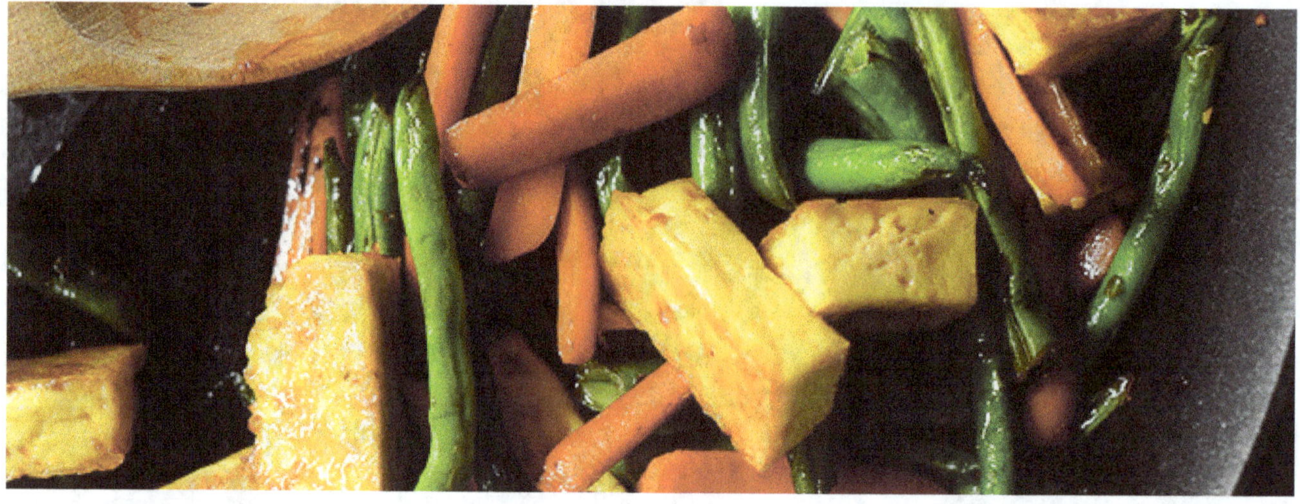

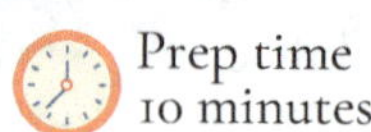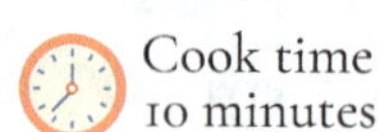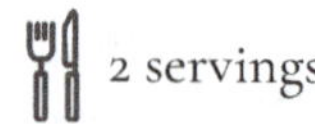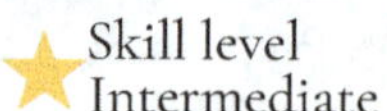

Tofu Stir- Fry

LUNCH

INGREDIENTS

1 block of firm tofu, pressed and cubed

1 cup broccoli florets

1 bell pepper, sliced

1 carrot, julienned

2 tablespoons soy sauce

1 tablespoon sesame oil

1 tablespoon olive oil

1 clove garlic, minced

NUTRITIONAL FACTS

Calories: 250

Protein: 15g

Carbohydrates: 15g

Fat: 15g

INSTRUCTIONS

1. Heat olive oil in a pan over medium heat.
2. Add tofu and cook until golden brown, then remove from the pan.
3. In the same pan, add sesame oil and garlic, and sauté for 1 minute.
4. Add broccoli, bell pepper, and carrot, and stir-fry until tender-crisp.
5. Return tofu to the pan, add soy sauce, and stir well to combine.

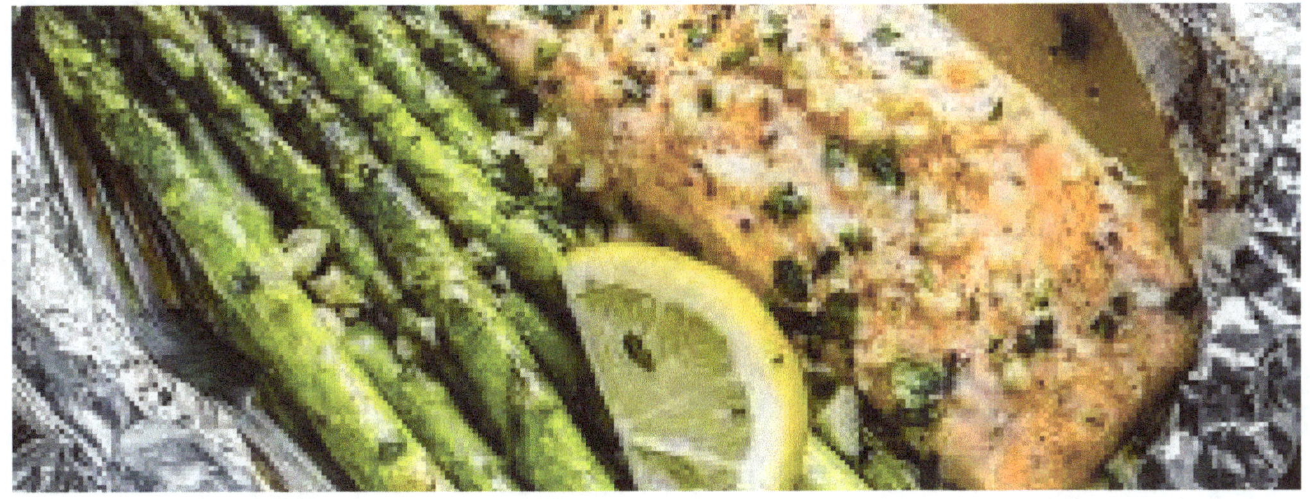

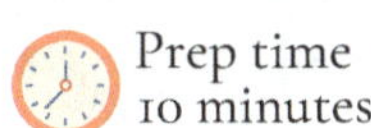 Prep time
10 minutes

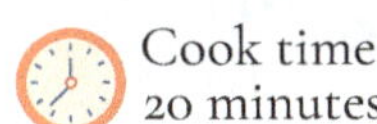 Cook time
20 minutes

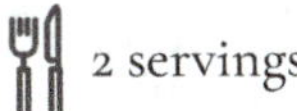 2 servings

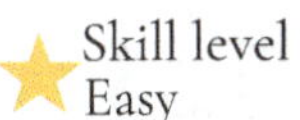 Skill level
Easy

Baked Salmon with Asparagus

DINNER

INGREDIENTS

2 salmon fillets

1 bunch asparagus, trimmed

2 tablespoons olive oil

1 lemon, sliced

Salt and pepper to taste

NUTRITIONAL FACTS

Calories: 300

Protein: 25g

Carbohydrates: 18g

Fat: 8g

INSTRUCTIONS

1. Preheat the oven to 400°F or (200°C).
2. Place the salmon fillets and asparagus on a baking sheet.
3. Drizzle with olive oil, then season with salt and pepper.
4. Arrange lemon slices on top.
5. Bake for 15-20 minutes, till salmon is cooked through.

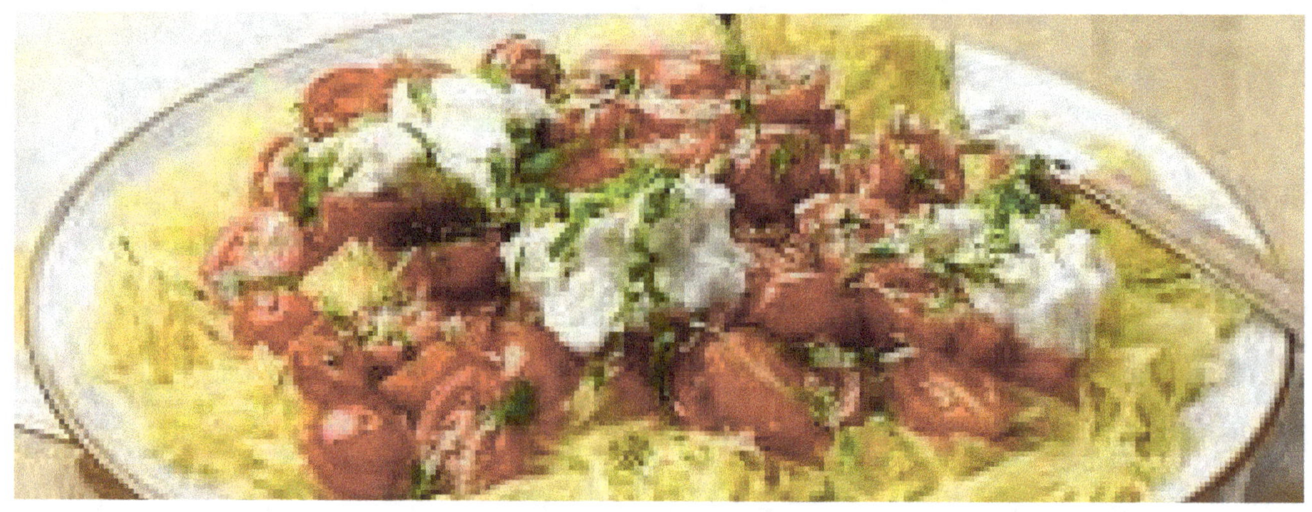

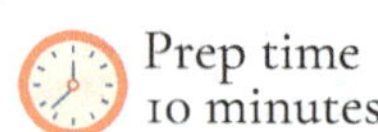 Prep time
10 minutes

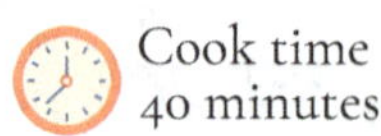 Cook time
40 minutes

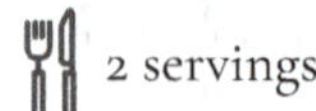 2 servings

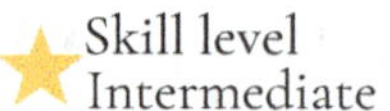 Skill level
Intermediate

Spaghetti Squash with Tomato Basil Sauce

DINNER

INGREDIENTS

1 spaghetti squash

2 tablespoons olive oil

1 can (14 oz) diced tomatoes

2 cloves garlic, minced

1/4 cup fresh basil, chopped

Salt and pepper to taste

NUTRITIONAL FACTS

Calories: 150

Protein: 3g

Carbohydrates: 25g

Fat: 5g

INSTRUCTIONS

1. Preheat oven to 400°F (200°C).

2. Cut spaghetti squash in half lengthwise, remove seeds, and drizzle with olive oil.

3. Place cut side down on a baking sheet and bake for 40 minutes.

4. In a pan, heat olive oil and sauté garlic until fragrant.

5. Add diced tomatoes and cook until heated through. Stir in basil.

6. Scrape spaghetti squash with a fork to create strands, and top with tomato basil sauce.

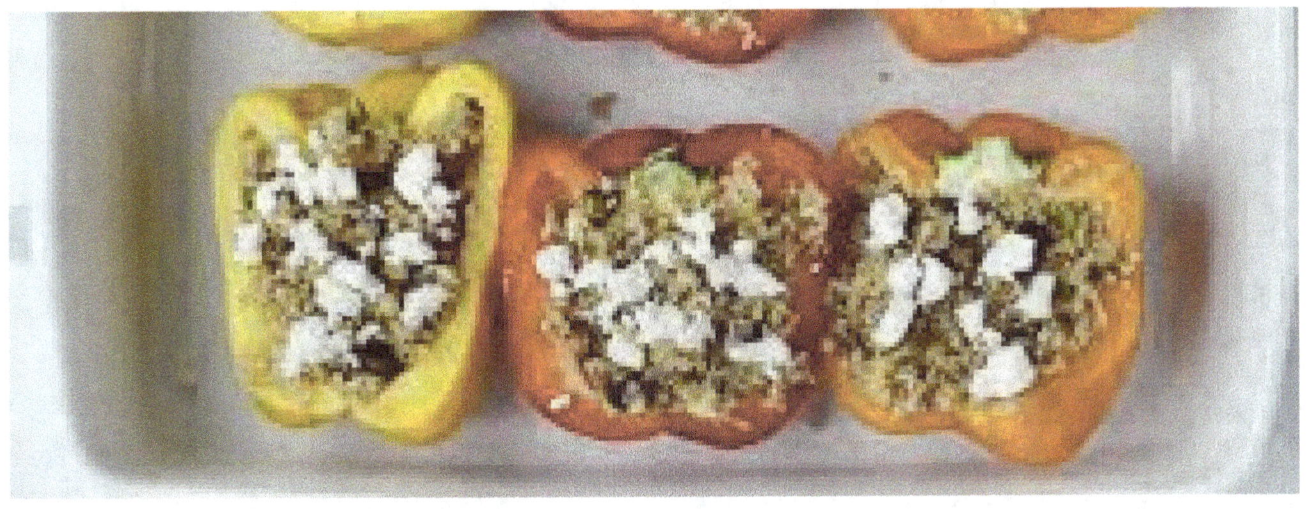

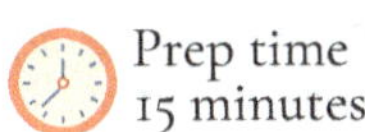
Prep time
15 minutes

Cook time
30 minutes

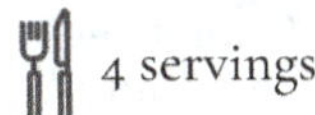
4 servings

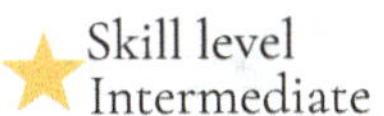
Skill level
Intermediate

Quinoa - Stuffed Bell Peppers

DINNER

INGREDIENTS

4 bell peppers, tops cut off and
seeds removed

1 cup cooked quinoa

1 can (15 oz) black beans,
drained and rinsed

1 cup corn kernels

1 cup diced tomatoes

1 teaspoon cumin

1 teaspoon chili powder

Salt and pepper to taste

NUTRITIONAL FACTS

Calories: 200

Protein: 8g

Carbohydrates: 35g

Fat: 3g

INSTRUCTIONS

1. Preheat oven to 375°F (190°C).
2. In a large bowl, mix quinoa, black beans, corn, tomatoes, cumin, and chili powder. Season with salt and pepper.
3. Stuff the bell peppers with the quinoa mixture and place in a baking dish.
4. Bake for 25-30 minutes, until peppers are tender.

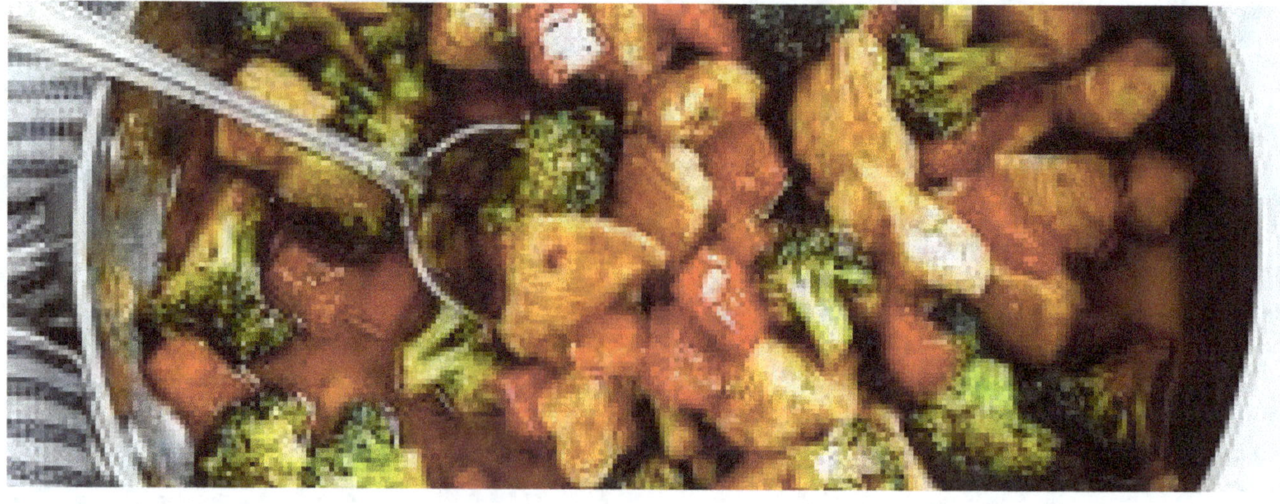

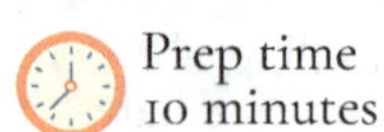
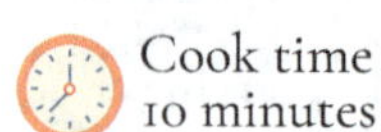
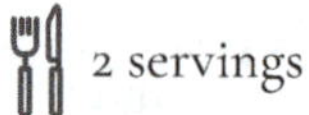
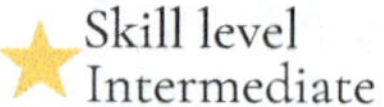

| Prep time 10 minutes | Cook time 10 minutes | 2 servings | Skill level Intermediate |

Chicken and Broccoli Stir - fry

DINNER

INGREDIENTS

2 chicken breasts, sliced thinly

2 cups broccoli florets

1 bell pepper, sliced

1 carrot, sliced

2 tablespoons soy sauce

1 tablespoon sesame oil

1 tablespoon olive oil

2 cloves garlic, minced

NUTRITIONAL FACTS

Calories: 300

Protein: 25g

Carbohydrates: 15g

Fat: 15g

INSTRUCTIONS

1. In a large pan, heat olive oil over medium heat.
2. Add chicken and cook until no longer pink, then remove from pan.
3. In the same pan, add sesame oil and garlic, and sauté for 1 minute.
4. Add broccoli, bell pepper, and carrot, and stir-fry until tender-crisp.
5. Return chicken to the pan, add soy sauce, and stir well to combine.

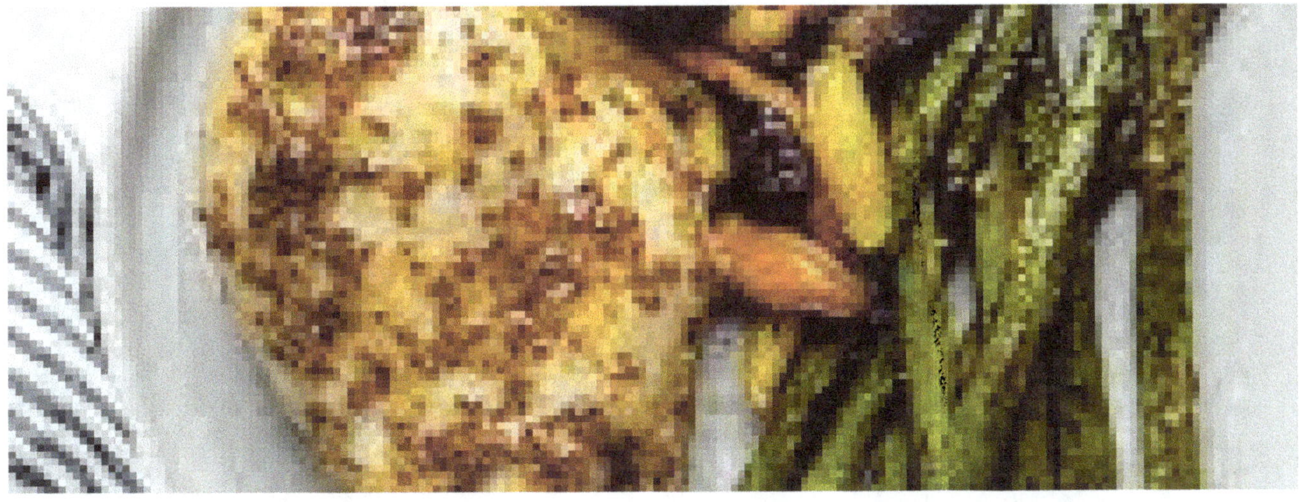

 Prep time
5 minutes

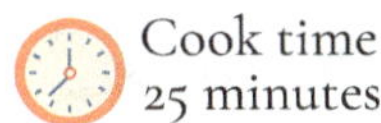 Cook time
25 minutes

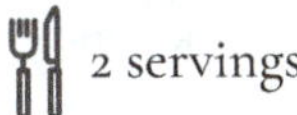 2 servings

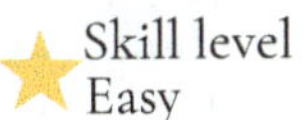 Skill level
Easy

Baked Chicken Breast

INGREDIENTS

2 boneless, skinless chicken breasts

2 tablespoons olive oil

1 teaspoon garlic powder

1 teaspoon paprika

Salt and pepper to taste

NUTRITIONAL FACTS

Calories: 220

Protein: 25g

Carbohydrates: -

Fat: 12g

INSTRUCTIONS

1. Preheat oven to 375°F (190°C).
2. Rub chicken breasts with olive oil, garlic powder, paprika, salt, and pepper.
3. Place chicken breasts in a baking dish and bake for 25-30 minutes, until cooked through.

DINNER

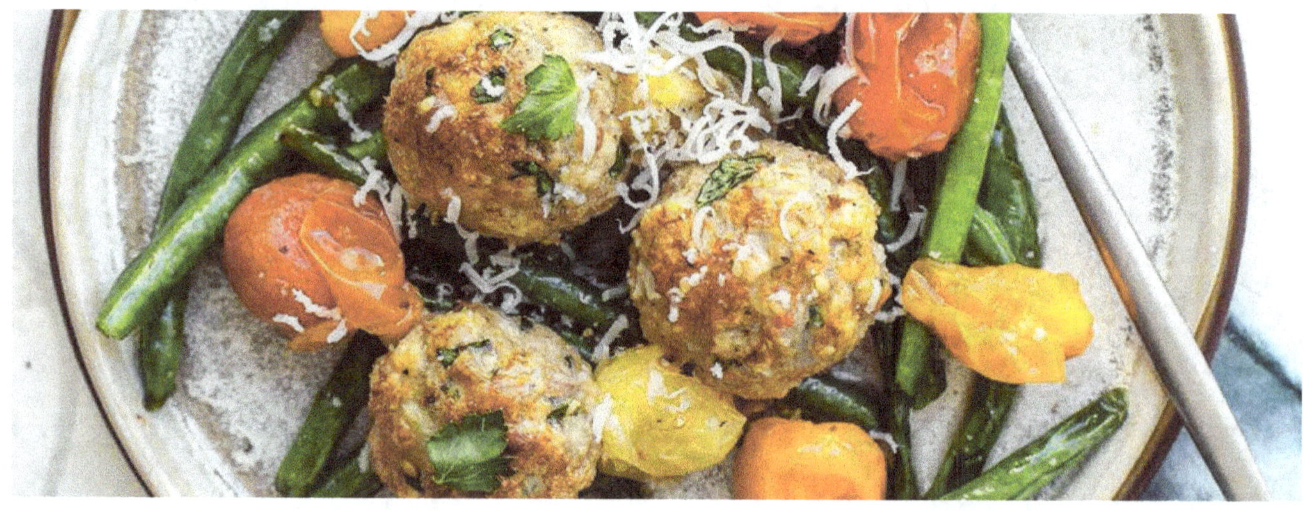

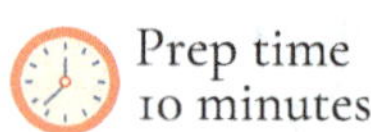 **Prep time**
10 minutes

 **Cook time**
25 minutes

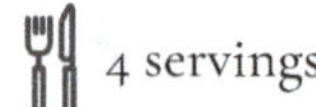 4 servings

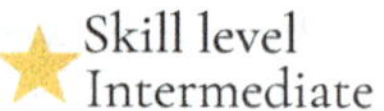 **Skill level**
Intermediate

Turkey Meat Balls

DINNER

INGREDIENTS

1 lb ground turkey

1/4 cup breadcrumbs

1 egg

1/4 cup grated Parmesan cheese

1 clove garlic, minced

1 teaspoon Italian seasoning

Salt and pepper to taste

INSTRUCTIONS

1. Preheat oven to 375°F (190°C).
2. In a large bowl, combine ground turkey, breadcrumbs, egg, Parmesan cheese, garlic, Italian seasoning, salt, and pepper.
3. Form the mixture into meatballs and place on a baking sheet.
4. Bake for 20-25 minutes, till cooked through.

NUTRITIONAL FACTS

Calories: 180

Protein: 20g

Carbohydrates: 5g

Fat: 9g

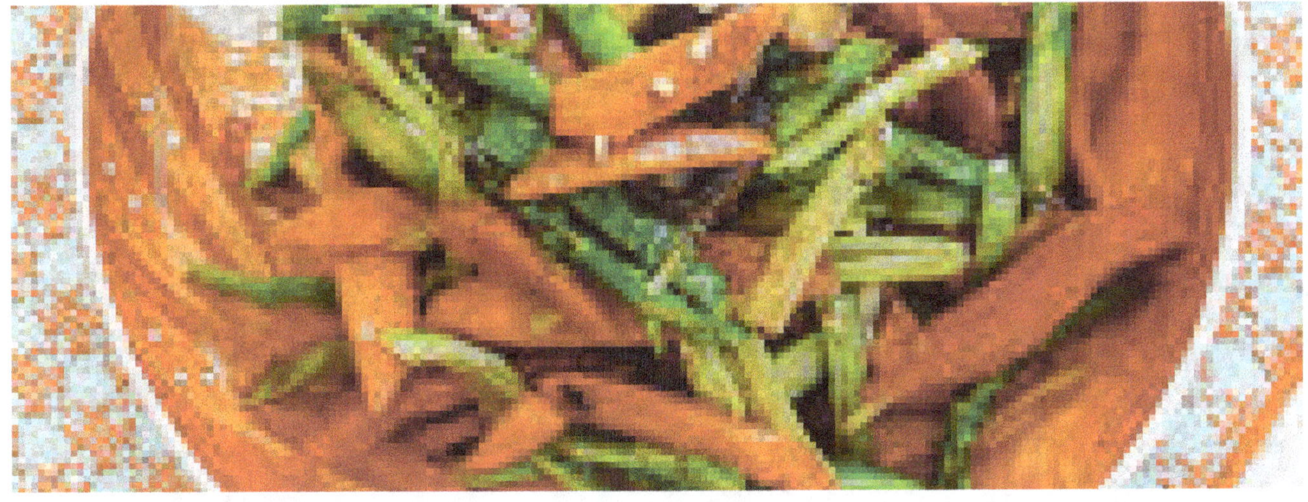

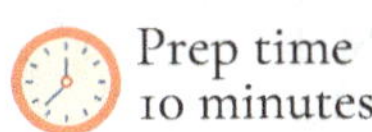 Prep time
10 minutes

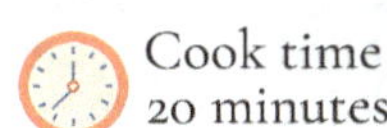 Cook time
20 minutes

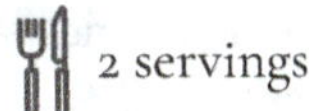 2 servings

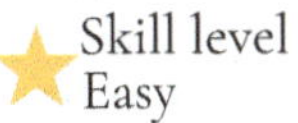 Skill level
Easy

Vegetable Stir - fry

INGREDIENTS

- 1 cup broccoli florets
- 1 bell pepper, sliced
- 1 carrot, sliced
- 1 cup snap peas
- 2 tablespoons soy sauce
- 1 tablespoon sesame oil
- 1 tablespoon olive oil
- 2 cloves garlic, minced

NUTRITIONAL FACTS

Calories: 150

Protein: 5g

Carbohydrates: 20g

Fat: 8g

INSTRUCTIONS

1. In a large pan, heat olive oil over medium heat.
2. Add garlic and sauté for a minute.
3. Add broccoli, bell pepper, carrot, and snap peas, and stir-fry until tender-crisp.
4. Add sesame oil and soy sauce, and stir well to combine.

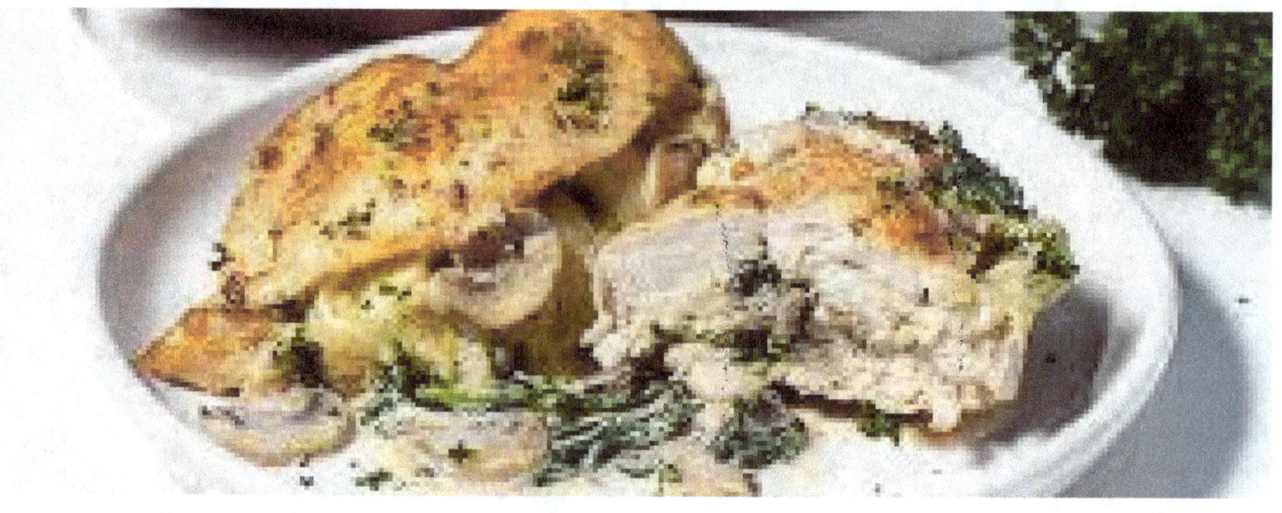

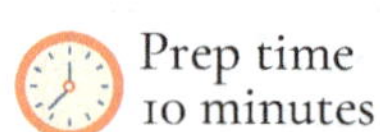 Prep time
10 minutes

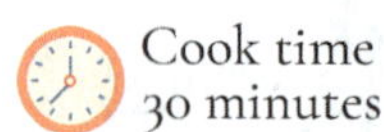 Cook time
30 minutes

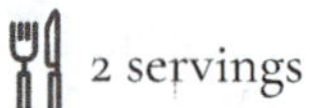 2 servings

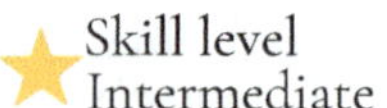 Skill level
Intermediate

Spinach & Mushroom Stuffed Chicken

INGREDIENTS

2 boneless, skinless chicken breasts

1 cup spinach leaves

1/2 cup sliced mushrooms

1/4 cup shredded mozzarella cheese

2 tablespoons olive oil

1 clove garlic, minced

Salt and pepper to taste

NUTRITIONAL FACTS

Calories: 300

Protein: 25g

Carbohydrates: 5g

Fat: 18g

INSTRUCTIONS

1. Preheat oven to 375°F (190°C).
2. In a pan, heat 1 tablespoon of olive oil and sauté garlic until fragrant.
3. Add spinach and mushrooms, and cook until wilted and tender.
4. Cut a pocket in each chicken breast and stuff with the spinach-mushroom mixture and mozzarella cheese.
5. Secure with toothpicks if needed.
6. Rub the chicken with the remaining olive oil, and season with salt and pepper.
7. Place in a baking dish and bake for 25-30 minutes, until chicken is cooked through.

DINNER

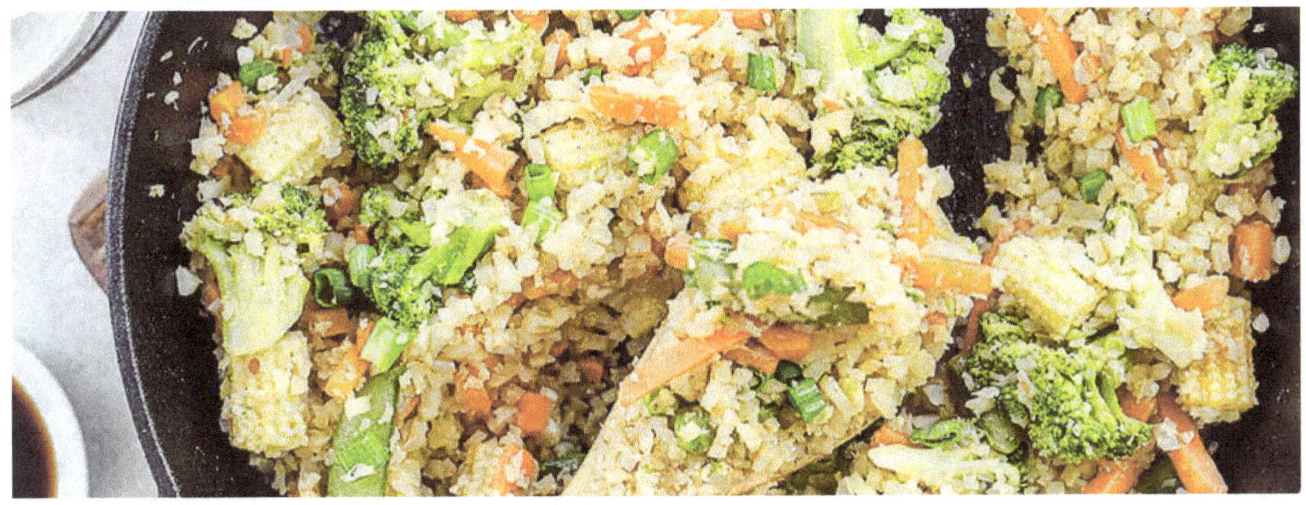

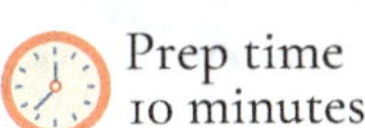 Prep time
10 minutes

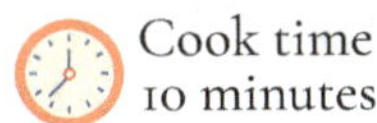 Cook time
10 minutes

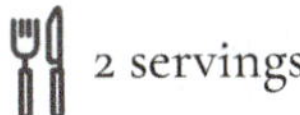 2 servings

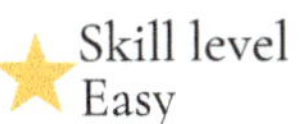 Skill level
Easy

Cauliflower Rice Stir-Fry

INGREDIENTS

1 head cauliflower, grated into rice-sized pieces

1 cup of mixed vegetables (carrots, peas, corn)

2 tablespoons soy sauce

1 tablespoon sesame oil

1 clove garlic, minced

1 tablespoon olive oil

NUTRITIONAL FACTS

Calories: 150

Protein: 3g

Carbohydrates: 15g

Fat: 9g

INSTRUCTIONS

1. In a large pan, heat olive oil over medium heat.
2. Add garlic and sauté for a minute.
3. Add mixed vegetables and cook until tender.
4. Add grated cauliflower and stir-fry until tender, about 5 minutes.
5. Add soy sauce and sesame oil, and stir well to combine.

DINNER

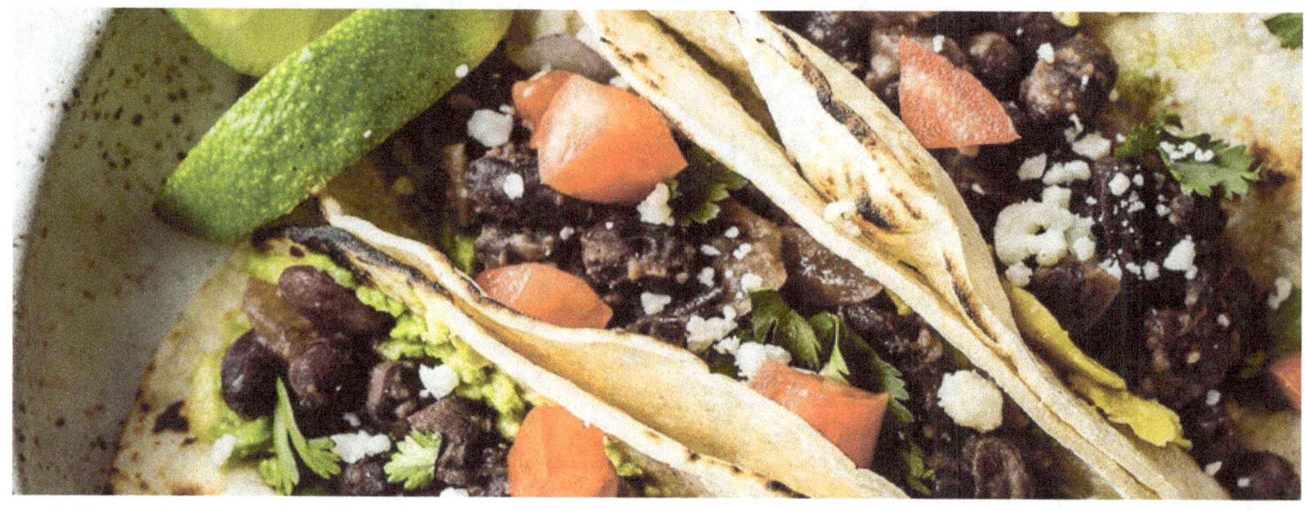

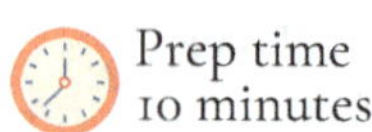 **Prep time**
10 minutes

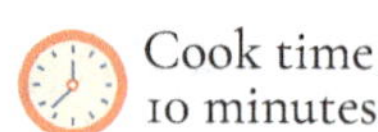 **Cook time**
10 minutes

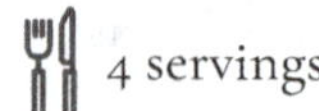 4 servings

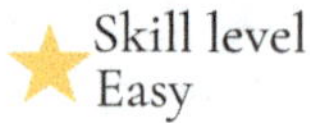 **Skill level**
Easy

Black Bean Tacos

INGREDIENTS

1 can (15 oz) of black beans, tired and rinsed

1 teaspoon cumin

1 teaspoon chili powder

1 tablespoon olive oil

8 small corn tortillas

1 cup shredded lettuce

1/2 cup diced tomatoes

1/4 cup diced red onion

1/4 cup chopped cilantro

1/4 cup crumbled feta cheese

NUTRITIONAL FACTS

Calories: 200

Protein: 8g

Carbohydrates: 30g

Fat: 5g

INSTRUCTIONS

1. In a large pan, heat olive oil over medium heat.
2. Add black beans, cumin, and chili powder, and cook until heated through.
3. Warm tortillas in a separate pan or microwave.
4. Assemble tacos by dividing black beans among tortillas, and topping with lettuce, tomatoes, red onion, cilantro, and feta cheese.

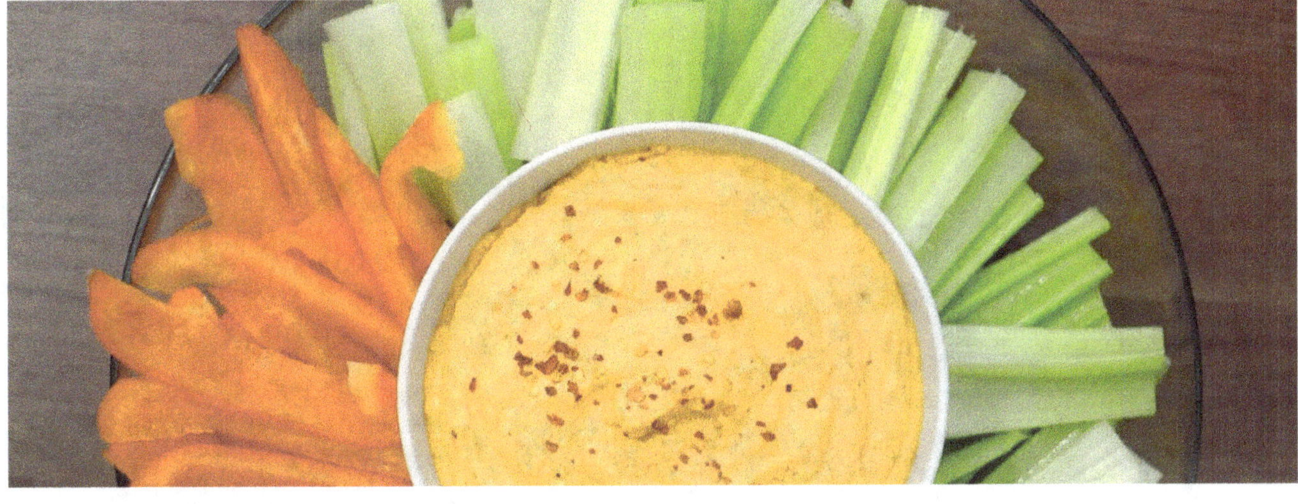

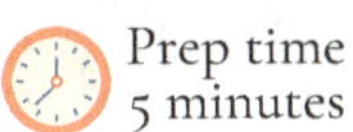 Prep time
5 minutes

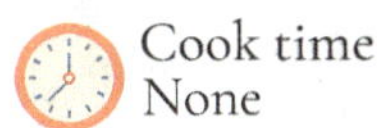 Cook time
None

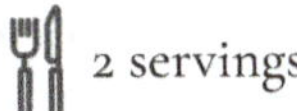 2 servings

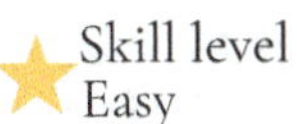 Skill level
Easy

Hummus and Veggie Sticks

INGREDIENTS

1 cup hummus

1 carrot, cut into sticks

1 cucumber, cut into sticks

1 bell pepper, cut into sticks

1 celery stalk, cut into sticks1

cup hummus

1 carrot, cut into sticks

1 cucumber, cut into sticks

1 bell pepper, cut into sticks

1 celery stalk, cut into sticks

NUTRITIONAL FACTS

Calories:150

Protein: 5g

Carbohydrates: 20g

Fat: 8g

INSTRUCTIONS

1. Arrange veggie sticks on a plate.

2. Serve with hummus for dipping.

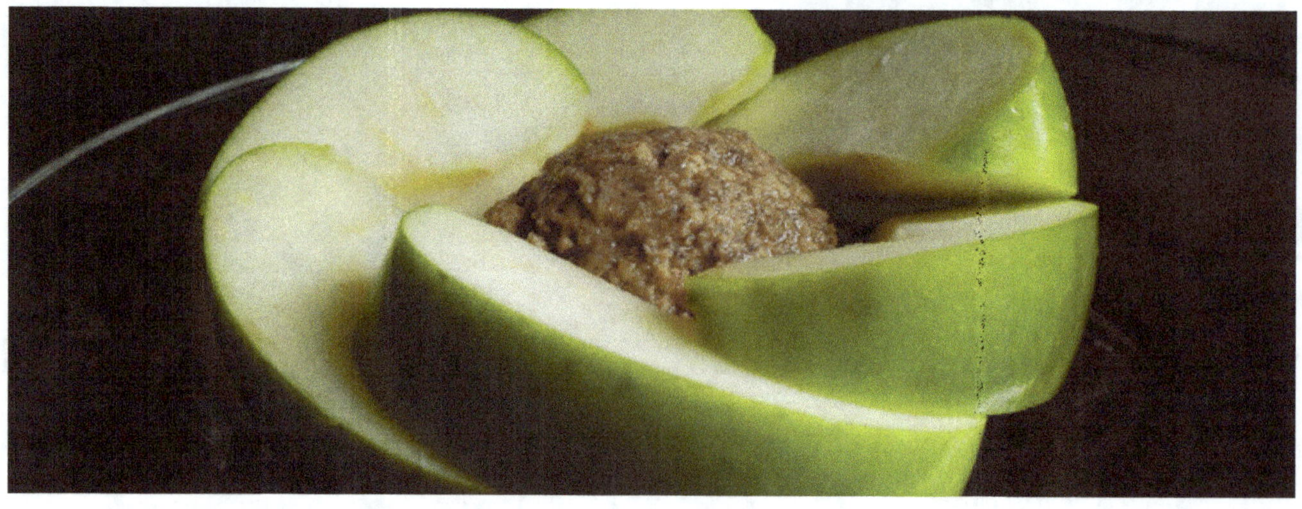

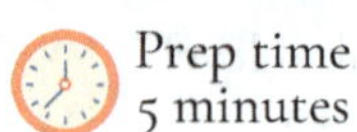 Prep time
5 minutes

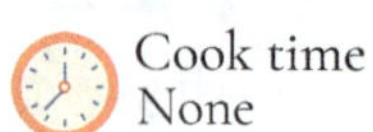 Cook time
None

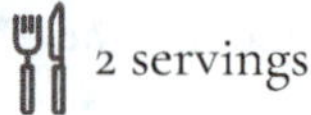 2 servings

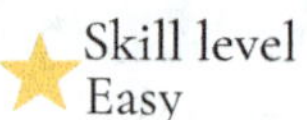 Skill level
Easy

Apple Slices with Almond Butter

INGREDIENTS

1 apple, sliced

2 tablespoons almond butter

NUTRITIONAL FACTS

Calories:200

Protein: 4g

Carbohydrates: 25g

Fat: 10g

INSTRUCTIONS

1. Arrange the apple slices on a plate.

2. Serve along with almond butter for dipping.

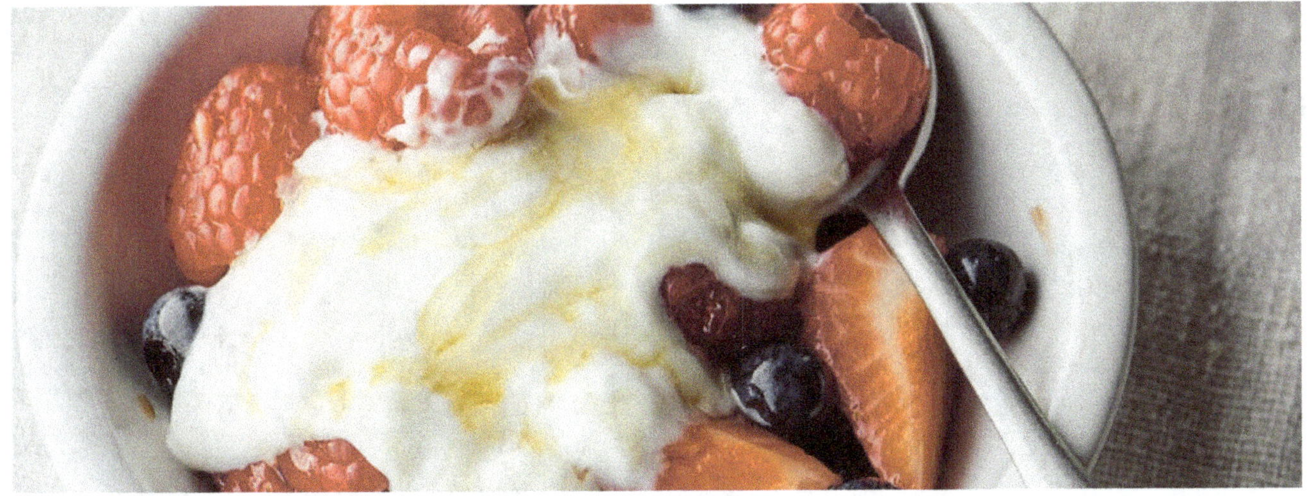

 Prep time
5 minutes

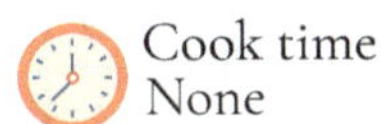 Cook time
None

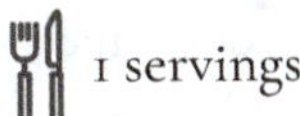 1 servings

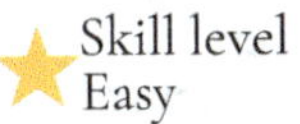 Skill level
Easy

Greek Yogurt with Berries

INGREDIENTS

1 cup Greek yogurt

1/2 cup mixed berries

1 tablespoon honey

INSTRUCTIONS

1. Spoon Greek yogurt into a bowl.

2. Top with mixed berries and drizzle with honey.

NUTRITIONAL FACTS

Calories:150

Protein: 12g

Carbohydrates: 20g

Fat: 2g

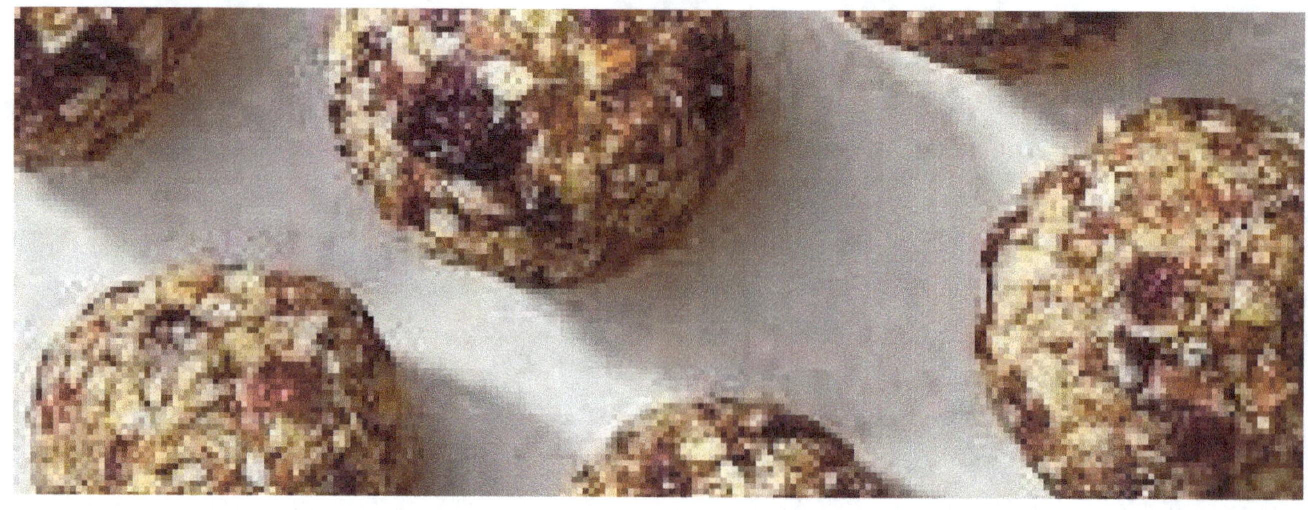

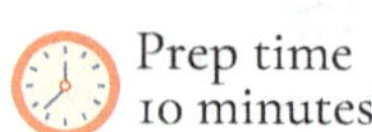 **Prep time**
10 minutes

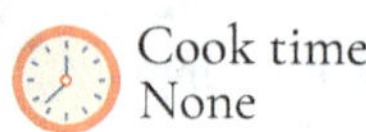 **Cook time**
None

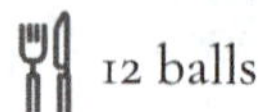 12 balls

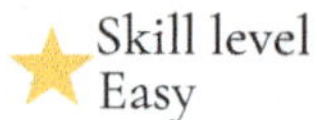 **Skill level**
Easy

Energy Balls

INGREDIENTS

1 cup rolled oats

1/2 cup peanut butter

1/4 cup honey

1/4 cup chocolate chips

NUTRITIONAL FACTS

Calories:100

Protein:3g

Carbohydrates: 15g

Fat: 5g

INSTRUCTIONS

1. In a bowl, mix together oats, peanut butter, honey, and chocolate chips.

2. Roll the mixture into small balls.

3. Refrigerate for at the least half-hour before being served.

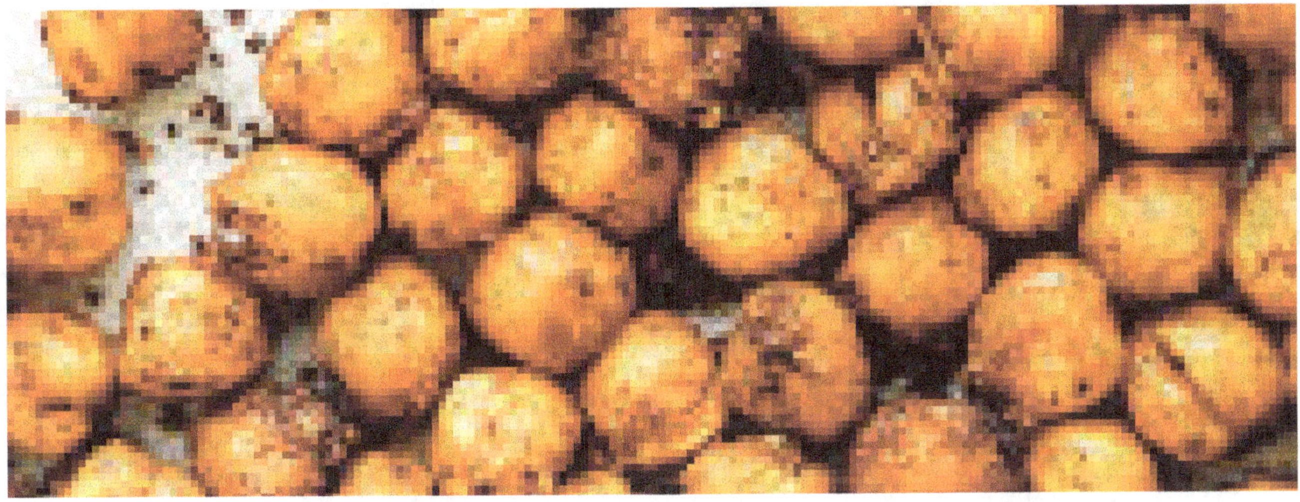

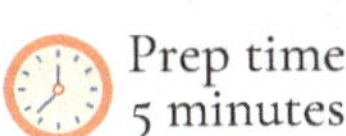
Prep time
5 minutes

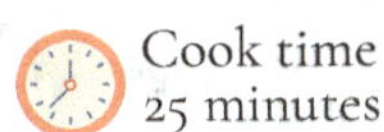
Cook time
25 minutes

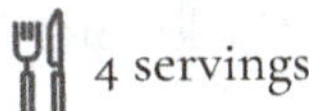
4 servings

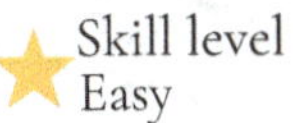
Skill level
Easy

Roasted Chickpeas

SNACKS

INGREDIENTS

1 can (15 oz) of chickpeas, tired and rinsed

1 tablespoon olive oil

1 teaspoon paprika

1 teaspoon garlic powder

Salt and pepper to taste

NUTRITIONAL FACTS

Calories:120

Protein: 5g

Carbohydrates: 20g

Fat: 3g

INSTRUCTIONS

1. Preheat oven to 400°F (200°C).

2. Toss chickpeas with olive oil, paprika, garlic powder, salt, and pepper.

3. Spread chickpeas on a baking sheet and roast for 20-25 minutes, until crispy.

Prep time
5 minutes

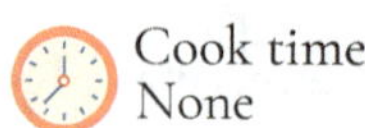
Cook time
None

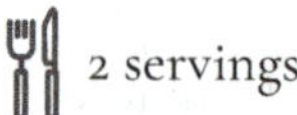
2 servings

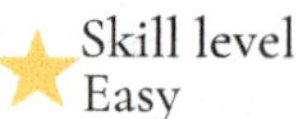
Skill level
Easy

Chia Seed Pudding with Mango

DESERTS

INGREDIENTS

1/4 cup chia seeds

1 cup almond milk

1 tablespoon honey

1/2 teaspoon vanilla extract

1/2 cup diced mango

NUTRITIONAL FACTS

Calories: 180

Protein: 4g

Carbohydrates: 25g

Fat: 8g

INSTRUCTIONS

1. In a bowl, combine chia seeds, almond milk, honey, and vanilla extract.
2. Stir well and refrigerate for at least 2 hours or overnight until thickened.
3. Top with diced mango before serving.

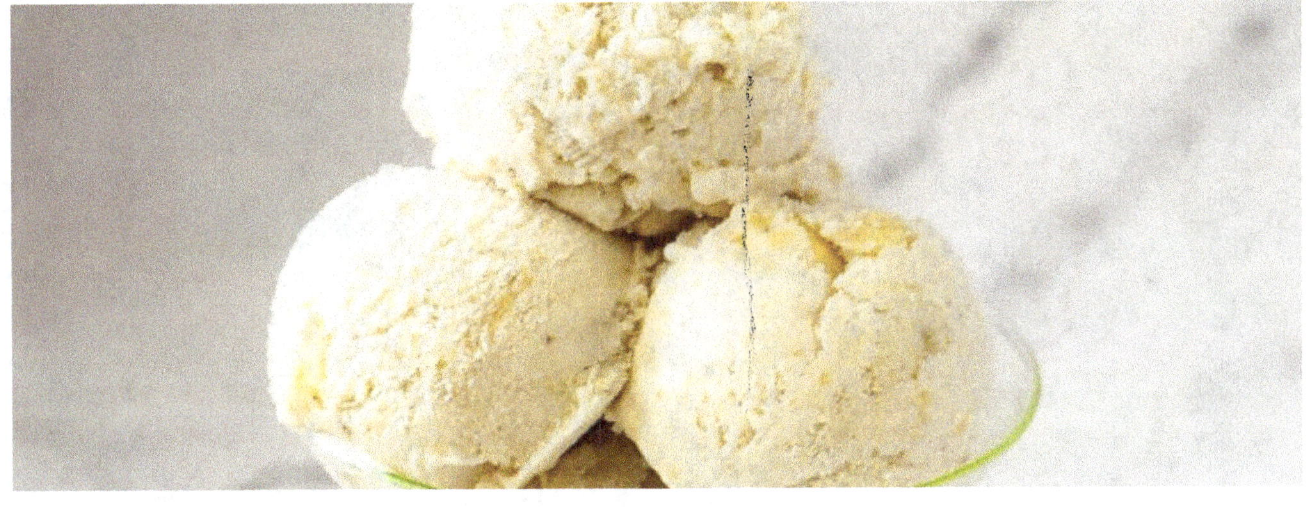

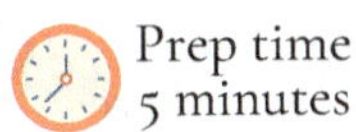 Prep time
5 minutes

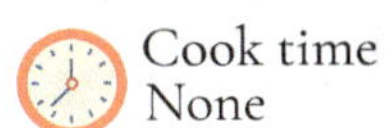 Cook time
None

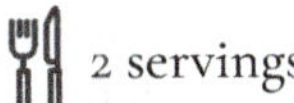 2 servings

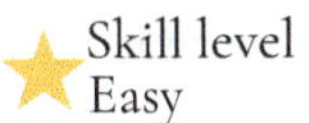 Skill level
Easy

Banana Ice Cream

DESERTS

INGREDIENTS

2 ripe bananas, sliced and frozen

1 teaspoon vanilla extract

NUTRITIONAL FACTS

Calories: 100

Protein: 1g

Carbohydrates: 25g

Fats: -

INSTRUCTIONS

1. Place frozen banana slices and vanilla extract in a blender.

2. Blend until smooth and creamy.

3. Serve immediately as soft serve or freeze for 1-2 hours for a firmer texture

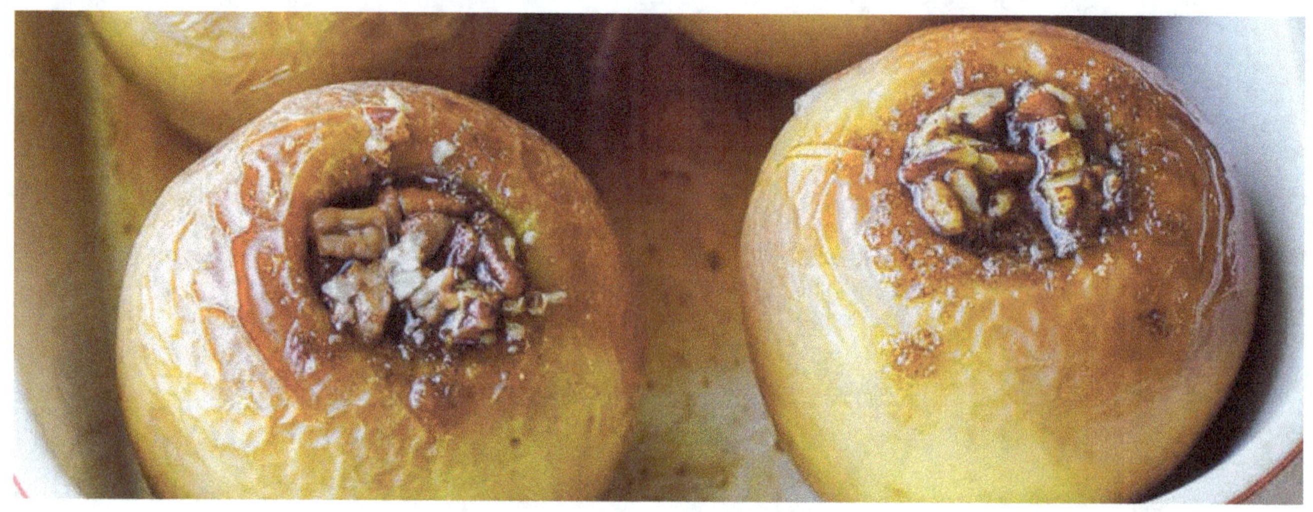

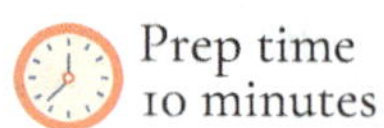
Prep time
10 minutes

Cook time
35 minutes

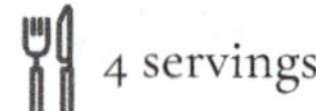
4 servings

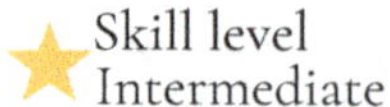
Skill level
Intermediate

Baked Apples

INGREDIENTS

DESERTS

4 apples, cored

1/4 cup rolled oats

2 tablespoons chopped nuts
(walnuts or pecans)

2 tablespoons raisins

1 teaspoon cinnamon

2 tablespoons honey

1/4 cup water

NUTRITIONAL FACTS

Calories: 150

Protein: 2g

Carbohydrates: 35g

Fat: 3g

INSTRUCTIONS

1. Preheat oven to 350°F (175°C).

2. In a bowl, mix oats, nuts, raisins, and cinnamon.

3. Stuff the apples with the oat mixture and place them in a baking dish.

4. Drizzle honey over the stuffed apples.

5. Pour water into the baking dish.

6. Bake for 30-35 minutes, until apples are tender

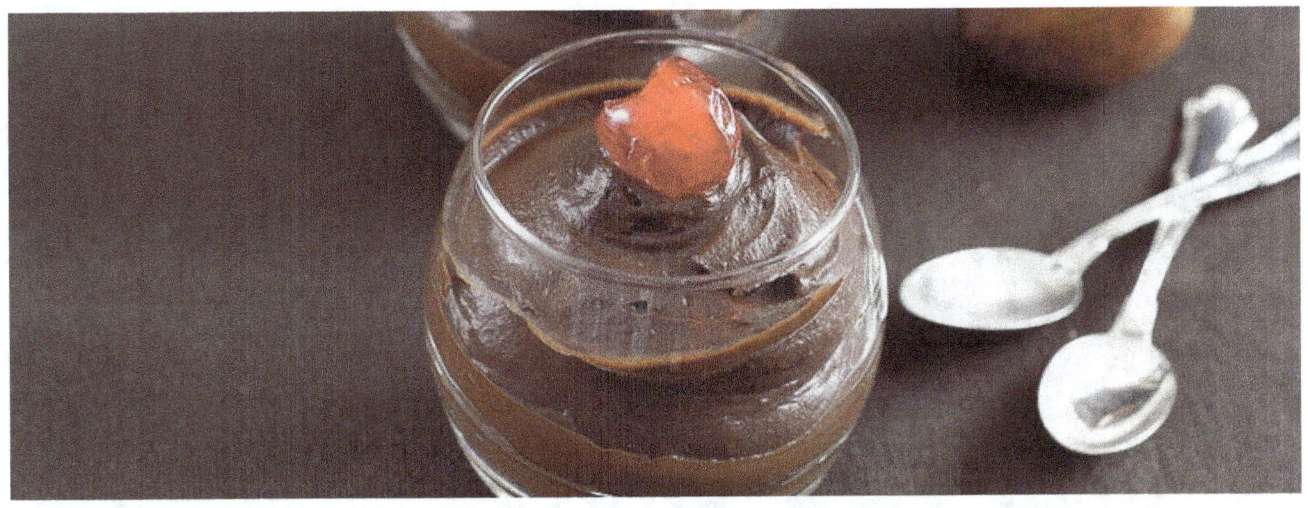

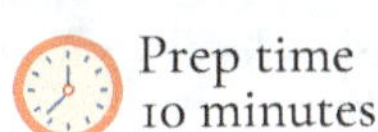
Prep time
10 minutes

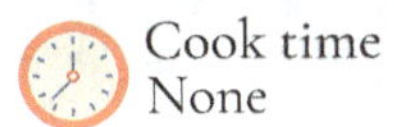
Cook time
None

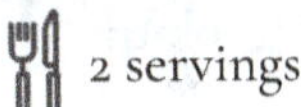
2 servings

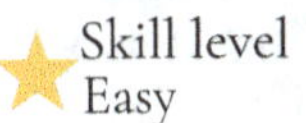
Skill level
Easy

Avocado Chocolate Mousse

DESERTS

INGREDIENTS

2 ripe avocados

1/4 cup cocoa powder

1/4 cup honey or maple syrup

1 teaspoon vanilla extract

Pinch of salt

INSTRUCTIONS

1. In a blender or food processor, combine avocados, cocoa powder, honey or maple syrup, vanilla extract, and salt.
2. Blend until smooth and creamy.
3. Refrigerate for at least half-hour before serving.

NUTRITIONAL FACTS

Calories: 200

Protein: 2g

Carbohydrates: 20g

Fats: 15g

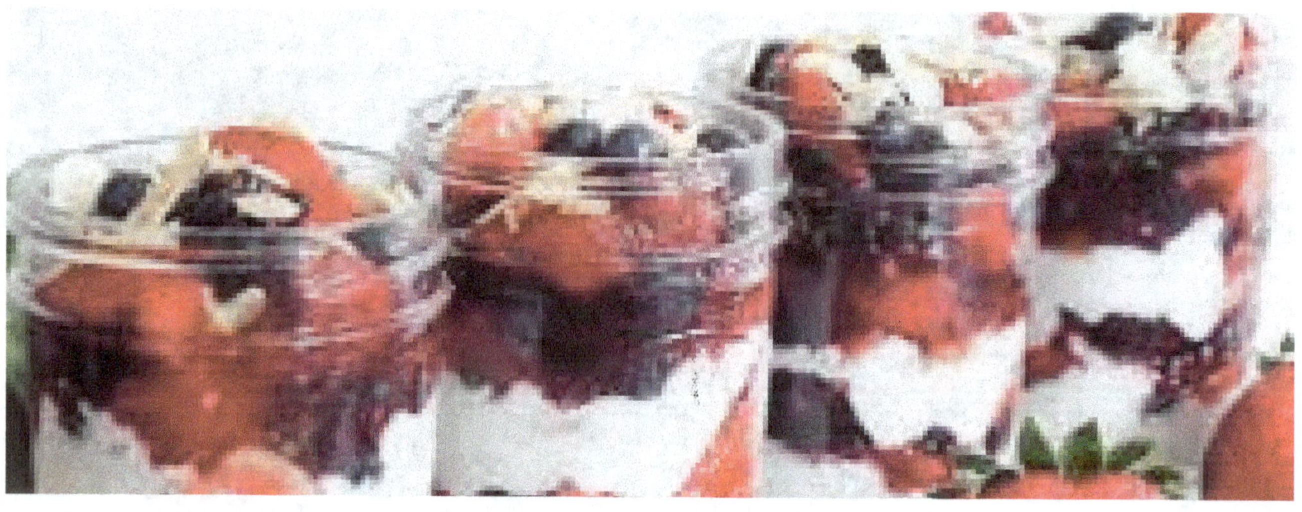

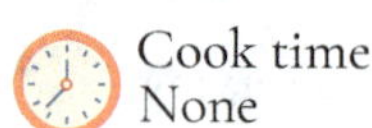

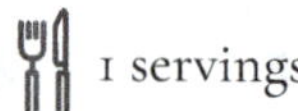

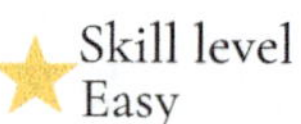

Berry Parfait

DESERTS

INGREDIENTS

1 cup Greek yogurt

1/2 cup mixed berries

1/4 cup granola

1 tablespoon honey

INSTRUCTIONS

1. In a glass or bowl, layer Greek yogurt, mixed berries, and granola.
2. Drizzle honey on top.

NUTRITIONAL FACTS

Calories: 200

Protein: 12g

Carbohydrates: 25g

Fat: 5g

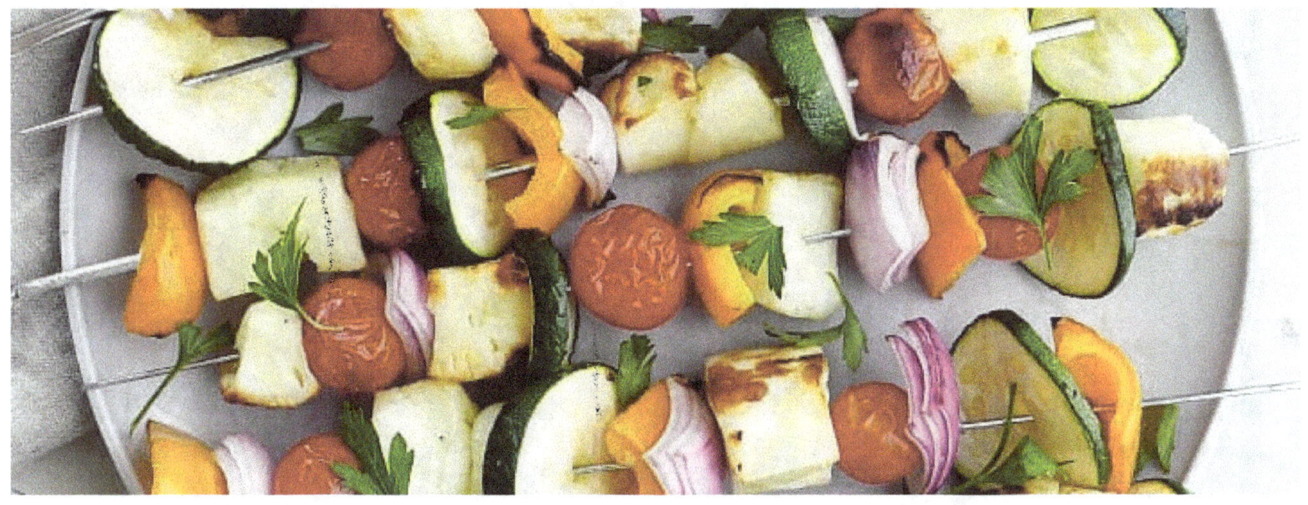

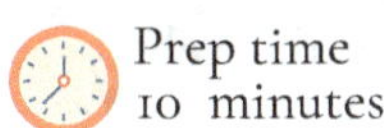
Prep time
10 minutes

Cook time
12 minutes

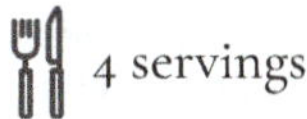
4 servings

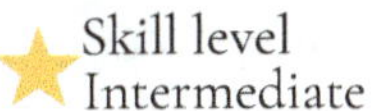
Skill level
Intermediate

Grilled Vegetable Skewers

INGREDIENTS

ADDITIONAL

1 zucchini, sliced

1 yellow squash, sliced

1 bell pepper, cut into chunks

1 red onion, cut into chunks

8 cherry tomatoes

2 tablespoons olive oil

1 teaspoon dried oregano

Salt and pepper to taste

NUTRITIONAL FACTS

Calories: 100

Protein: 2g

Carbohydrates: 15g

Fat: 5g

INSTRUCTIONS

1. Preheat grill to medium-high heat.
2. Thread zucchini, yellow squash, bell pepper, red onion, and cherry tomatoes onto skewers.
3. Brush with olive oil and sprinkle with oregano, salt, and pepper.
4. Grill for 10-12 minutes, turning occasionally, until vegetables are tender and slightly charred.

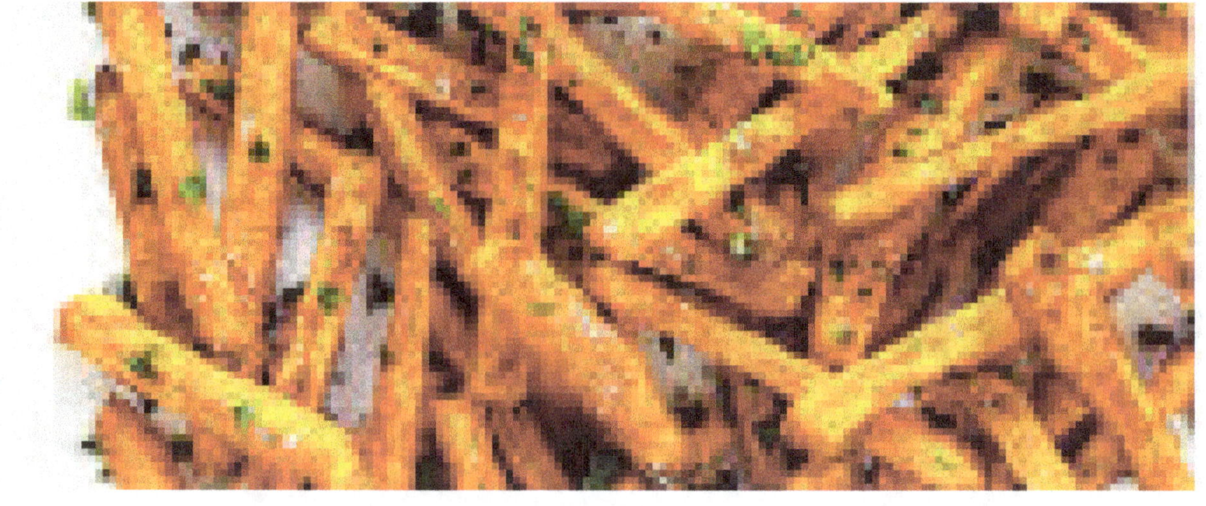

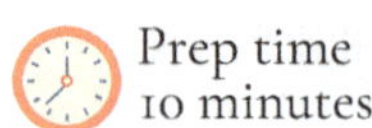 Prep time
10 minutes

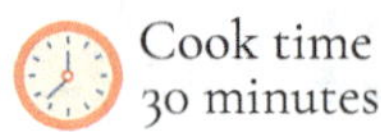 Cook time
30 minutes

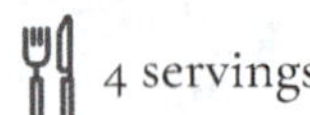 4 servings

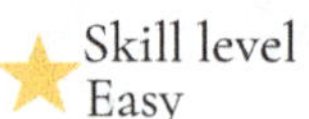 Skill level
Easy

Baked Sweet Potato Fries

INGREDIENTS

2 tablespoons olive oil

1 teaspoon paprika

1/2 teaspoon garlic powder

Salt and pepper to taste

NUTRITIONAL FACTS

Calories: 150

Protein: 2g

Carbohydrates: 30g

Fat: 5g

INSTRUCTIONS

1. Preheat oven to 425°F (220°C).

2. In a big bowl, toss sweet potato fries with olive oil, paprika, garlic powder, salt, and pepper.

3. Spread fries in a single layer on a baking sheet.

4. Bake for 25-30 minutes, flipping halfway through, until crispy and golden.

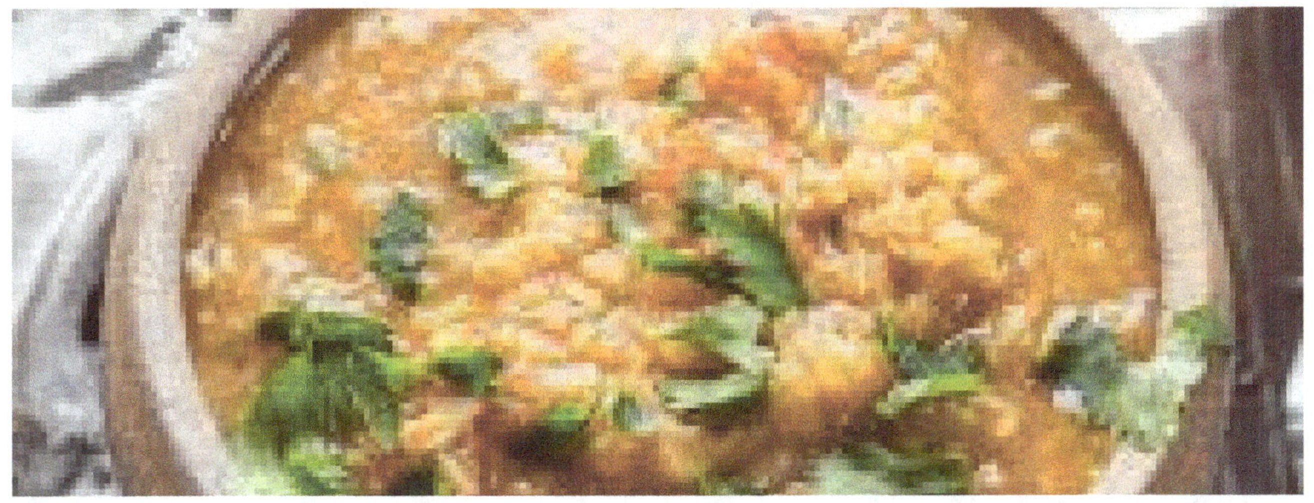

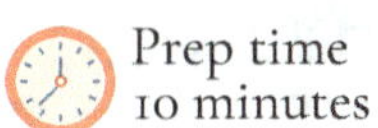
Prep time
10 minutes

Cook time
30 minutes

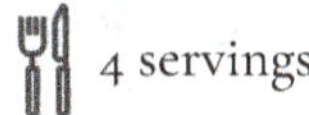
4 servings

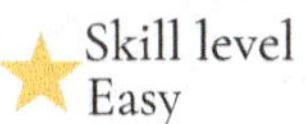
Skill level
Easy

Lentil Soup

INGREDIENTS

ADDITIONAL

1 cup lentils, rinsed

1 carrot, diced

1 celery stalk, diced

1 onion, chopped

2 cloves garlic, minced

4 cups vegetable broth

1 can (14 oz) diced tomatoes

1 teaspoon cumin

1 teaspoon paprika

2 tablespoons olive oil

Salt and pepper to taste

NUTRITIONAL FACTS

Calories: 250

Protein: 12g

Carbohydrates: 40g

Fat: 8g

INSTRUCTIONS

1. In a large pot, heat the olive oil over medium heat. Add onion, carrot, and celery, and cook until softened.

2. Add garlic, cumin, and paprika, and cook for 1 minute.

3. Add lentils, vegetable broth, and diced tomatoes. Bring to a boil.

4. Reduce heat and simmer for 30-35 minutes, until lentils are tender.

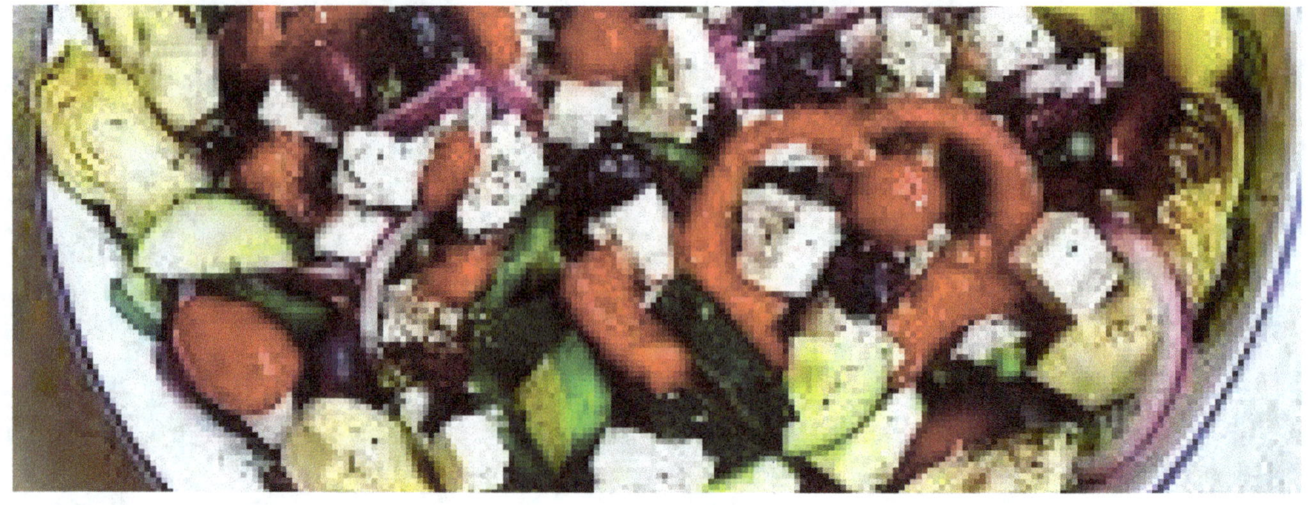

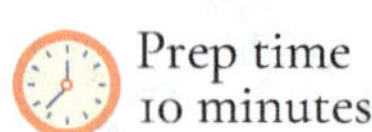
Prep time
10 minutes

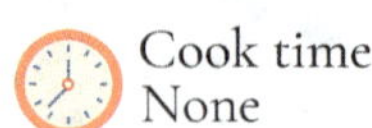
Cook time
None

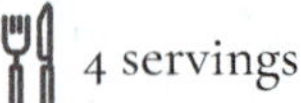
4 servings

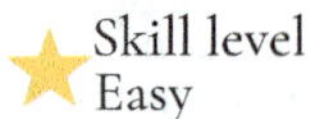
Skill level
Easy

Greek Salad

INGREDIENTS

ADDITIONAL

1 cucumber, diced

1 cup cherry tomatoes, halved

1/4 red onion, thinly sliced

1/2 cup Kalamata olives, pitted and halved

1/2 cup feta cheese, crumbled

NUTRITIONAL FACTS

Calories: 150

Protein: 5g

Carbohydrates: 10g

Fat: 10g

INSTRUCTIONS

1. In a large bowl, combine cucumber, cherry tomatoes, red onion, olives, and feta cheese.
2. In a small bowl, whisk the olive oil, wine vinegar, oregano, salt, and pepper.
3. Pour the dressing over the salad and toss to combine.

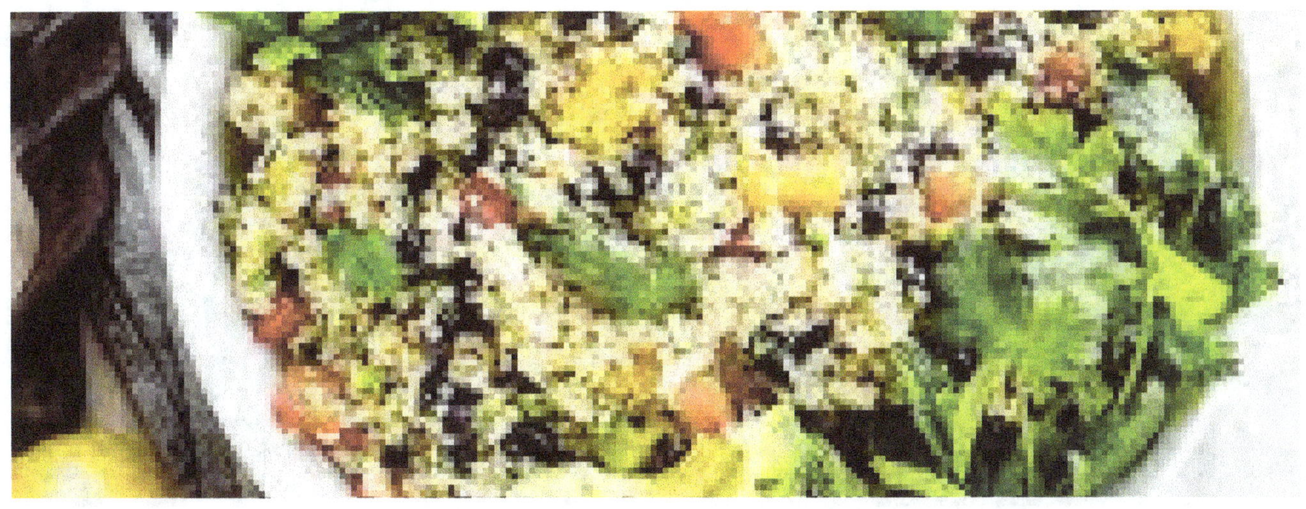

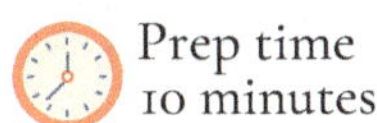
Prep time
10 minutes

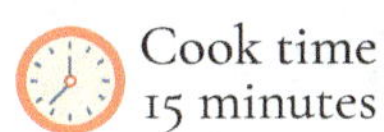
Cook time
15 minutes

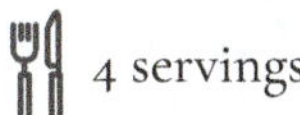
4 servings

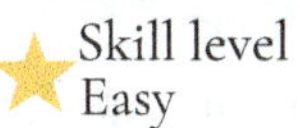
Skill level
Easy

Mango and Black Bean Quinoa Salad

INGREDIENTS

- 1 cup quinoa
- 2 cups water
- 1 can black beans, drained and rinsed
- 1 ripe mango, diced
- 1 red bell pepper, diced
- 1/4 cup chopped fresh cilantro
- 1/4 cup lime juice
- 2 tablespoons olive oil
- 1 teaspoon ground cumin
- Salt and pepper to taste

INSTRUCTIONS

1. Rinse quinoa under cold water. In a medium pot, bring water to a boil, add quinoa, cover, and reduce heat. Simmer for 15 minutes or until water is absorbed.
2. In a large bowl, combine cooked quinoa, black beans, mango, bell pepper, and cilantro.
3. In a small bowl, whisk together lime juice, olive oil, cumin, salt, and pepper. Pour over quinoa mixture and toss to coat.
4. Chill in the refrigerator for at least 30 minutes before serving.

NUTRITIONAL FACTS

- Calories: 250
- Protein: 8g
- Carbohydrates: 40g
- Fat: 7g

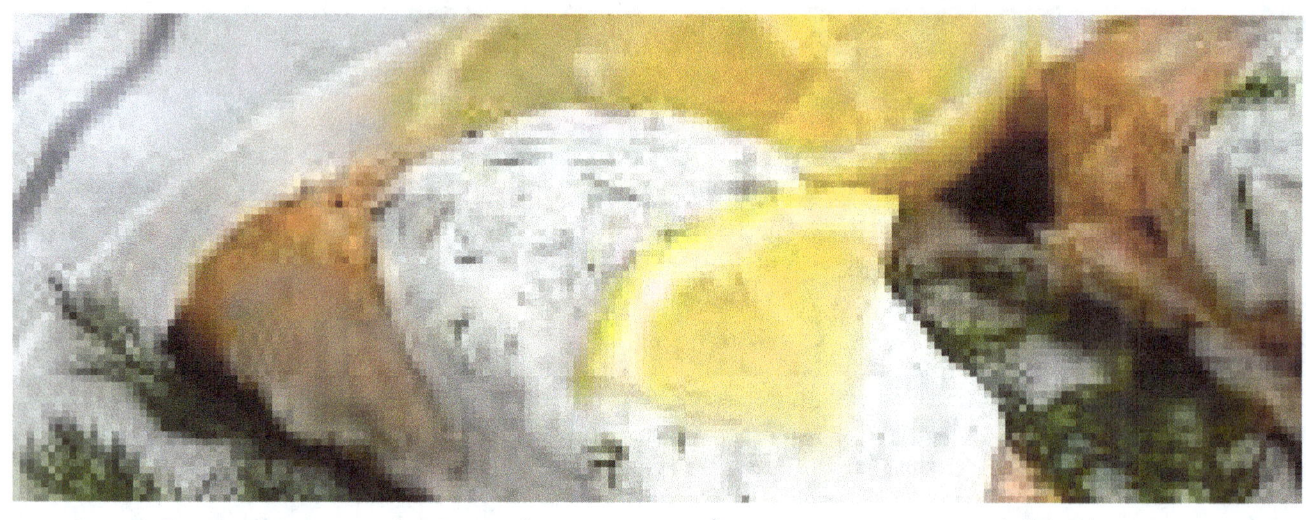

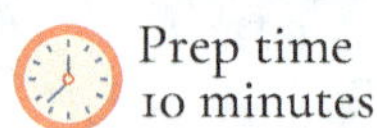
Prep time
10 minutes

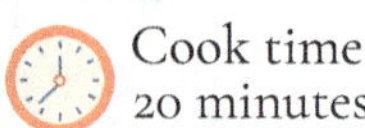
Cook time
20 minutes

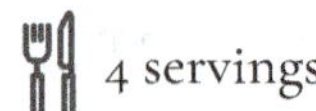
4 servings

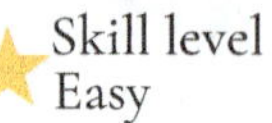
Skill level
Easy

Baked Salmon with Dill Sauce

INGREDIENTS

ADDITIONAL

- 4 salmon fillets
- 2 tablespoons olive oil
- Salt and pepper to taste
- 1/2 cup plain Greek yogurt
- 1 tablespoon fresh dill, chopped
- 1 tablespoon lemon juice
- 1 teaspoon lemon zest
- 1 clove garlic, minced

NUTRITIONAL FACTS

- Calories: 320
- Protein: 34g
- Carbohydrates: 2g
- Fat: 20g

INSTRUCTIONS

1. Preheat oven to 375°F (190°C). Line a baking sheet with parchment paper.
2. Place salmon fillets on the baking sheet, drizzle with olive oil, and season with salt and pepper.
3. Bake for 15-20 minutes, or until salmon flakes easily with a fork.
4. In a small bowl, mix Greek yogurt, dill, lemon juice, lemon zest, and garlic. Serve sauce over baked salmon.

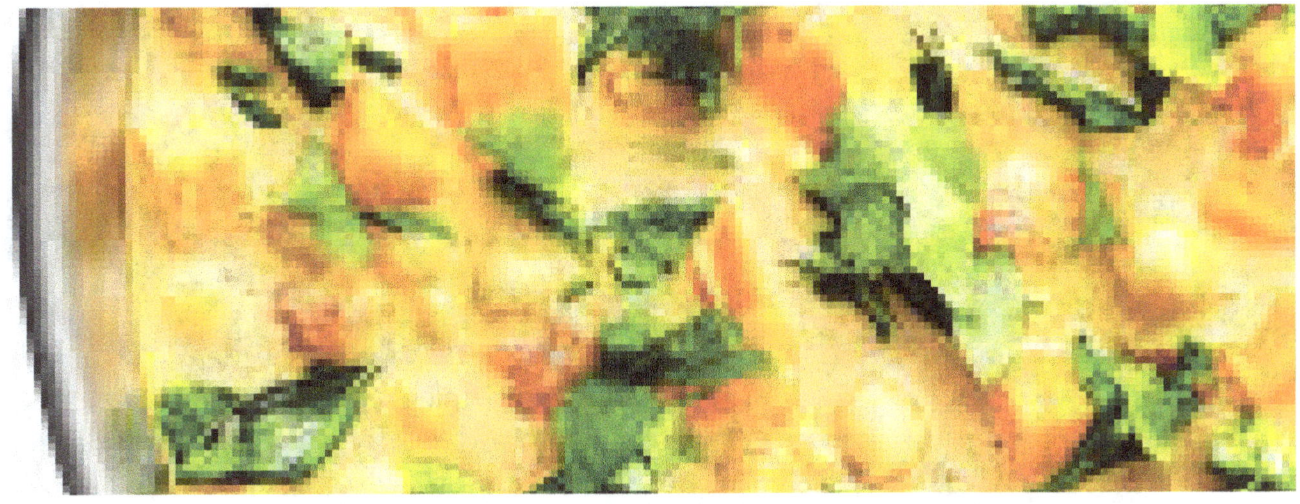

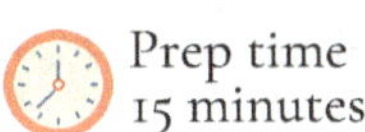
Prep time
15 minutes

Cook time
25 minutes

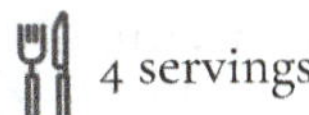
4 servings

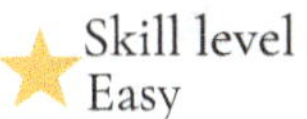
Skill level
Easy

Sweet Potato and Chickpea Curry

ADDITIONAL

INGREDIENTS

- 1 tablespoon grated ginger
- 2 teaspoons curry powder
- 1 teaspoon ground cumin
- 1 teaspoon ground turmeric
- 2 large sweet potatoes, peeled and cubed
- 1 can diced tomatoes
- 1 can coconut milk
- 1 can chickpeas, drained and rinsed
- Salt and pepper to taste
- Fresh cilantro for garnish

INSTRUCTIONS

1. Heat olive oil in a large pot over medium heat. Add onion, garlic, and ginger, and sauté until onion is translucent.
2. Add curry powder, cumin, and turmeric, and cook for 1 minute until fragrant.
3. Stir in sweet potatoes, tomatoes, coconut milk, and chickpeas. Season with salt and pepper.
4. Bring to a simmer, cover, and cook for 20-25 minutes, or until sweet potatoes are tender.
5. Garnish with fresh cilantro before serving.

NUTRITIONAL FACTS

- Calories: 350
- Protein: 8g
- Carbohydrates: 50g
- Fat: 14g

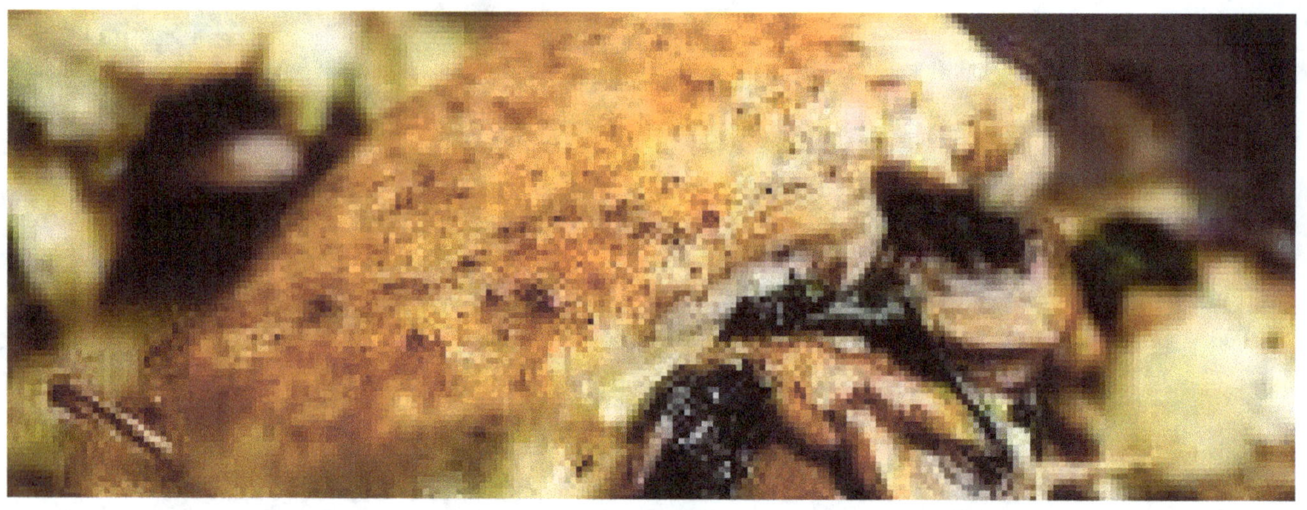

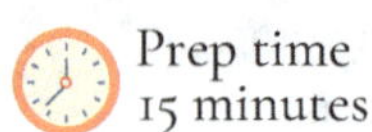
Prep time
15 minutes

Cook time
25 minutes

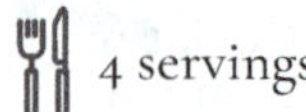
4 servings

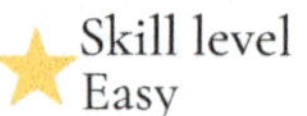
Skill level
Easy

Spinach and Mushroom Stuffed Chicken Breast

INGREDIENTS

ADDITIONAL

- 4 boneless, skinless chicken breasts
- 2 tablespoons olive oil
- 2 cups fresh spinach, chopped
- 1 cup mushrooms, diced
- 1/2 cup feta cheese, crumbled
- 1/2 teaspoon garlic powder
- Salt and pepper to taste
- Toothpicks or kitchen twine

NUTRITIONAL FACTS

- Calories: 300
- Protein: 34g
- Carbohydrates: 3g
- Fat: 16g

INSTRUCTIONS

1. Preheat oven to 375°F (190°C).
2. Heat 1 tablespoon of olive oil in a skillet over medium heat. Add spinach and mushrooms, and sauté until spinach is wilted and mushrooms are tender. Remove from heat and stir in feta cheese.
3. Cut a pocket in each chicken breast and stuff with spinach mixture. Secure with toothpicks or kitchen twine.
4. Heat remaining olive oil in an ovenproof skillet over medium-high heat. Sear chicken breasts for 2-3 minutes per side until golden brown.
5. Transfer skillet to the oven and bake for 20 minutes, or until chicken is cooked through.

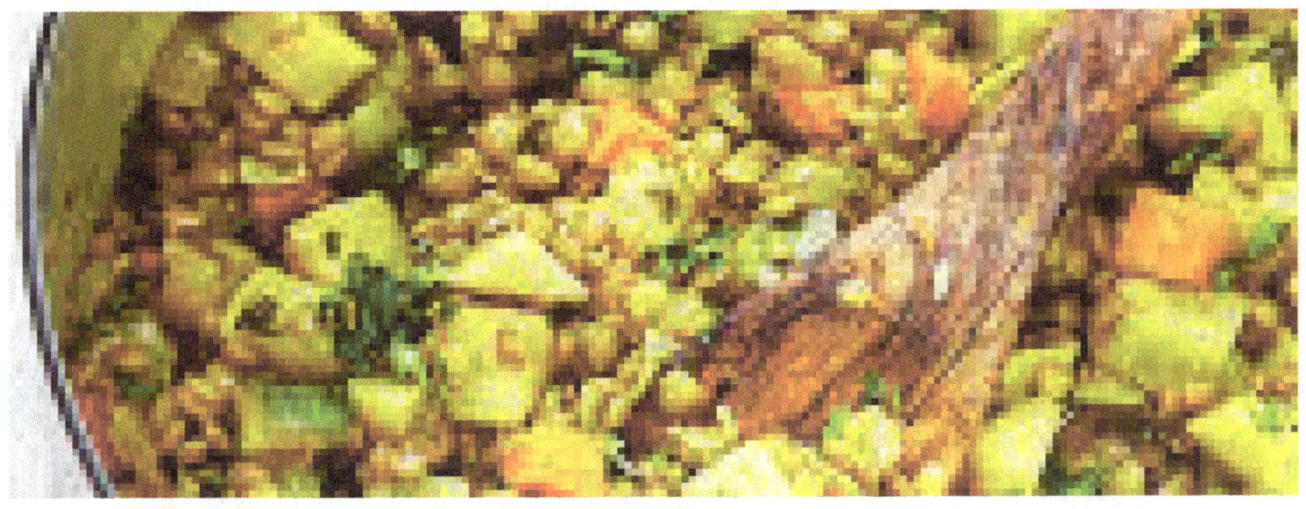

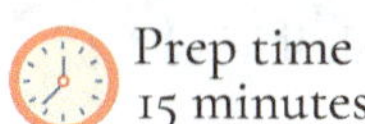 Prep time
15 minutes

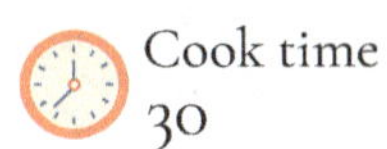 Cook time
30 minutes

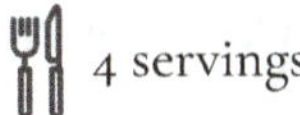 4 servings

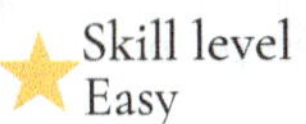 Skill level
Easy

Lentil and Vegetable Stew

INGREDIENTS

ADDITIONAL

- 2 tablespoons olive oil
- 1 onion, diced
- 2 carrots, sliced
- 2 celery stalks, sliced
- 3 cloves garlic, minced
- 1 cup dried lentils, rinsed
- 1 can diced tomatoes
- 4 cups vegetable broth
- 1 teaspoon dried thyme
- 1 teaspoon dried oregano
- 2 cups chopped kale
- Salt and pepper to taste

INSTRUCTIONS

1. Heat olive oil in a large pot over medium heat. Add onion, carrots, and celery, and sauté until vegetables are softened.
2. Add garlic and cook for 1 minute until fragrant.
3. Stir in lentils, tomatoes, broth, thyme, and oregano. Bring to a boil, then reduce heat and simmer for 25-30 minutes, or until lentils are tender.
4. Stir in kale and cook for 5 more minutes. Season with salt and pepper.

NUTRITIONAL FACTS

- Calories: 250
- Protein: 12g
- Carbohydrates: 40g
- Fat: 6g

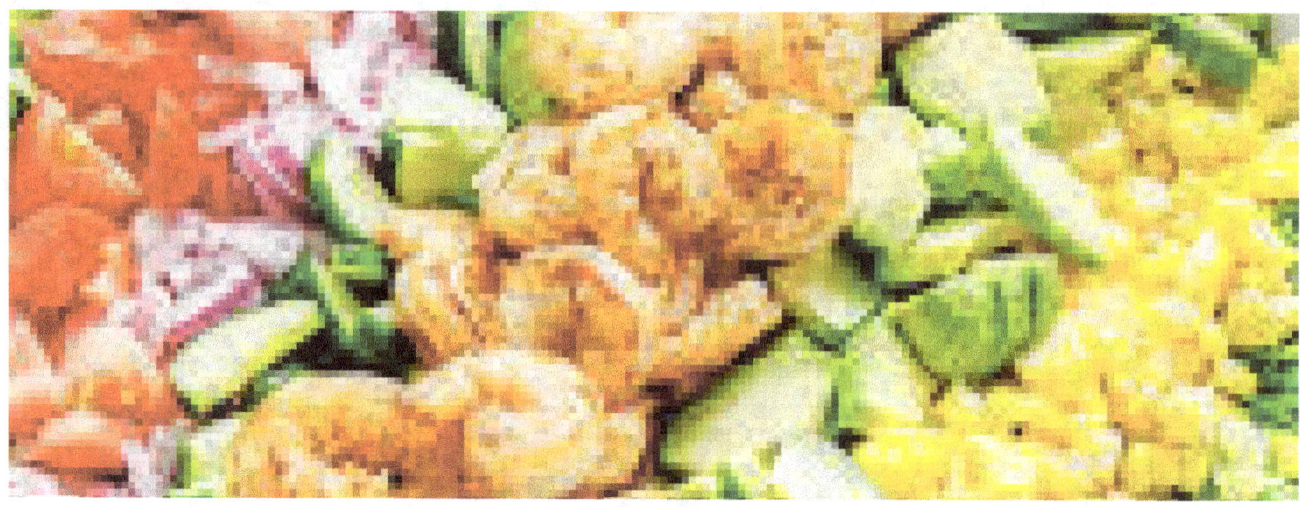

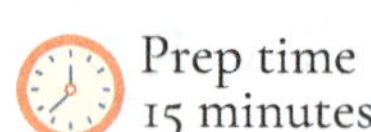 **Prep time**
15 minutes

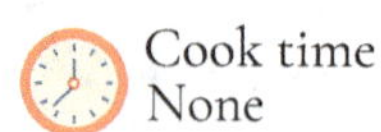 **Cook time**
None

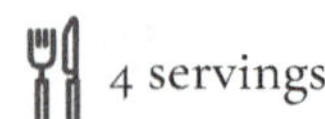 4 servings

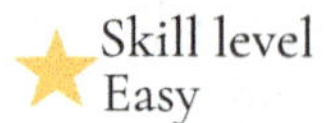 **Skill level**
Easy

Shrimp and Avocado Salad

INGREDIENTS

ADDITIONAL

- 1 lb cooked shrimp, peeled and deveined
- 2 avocados, diced
- 1 cup cherry tomatoes, halved
- 1/4 cup red onion, finely diced
- 2 tablespoons fresh lime juice
- 2 tablespoons olive oil
- Salt and pepper to taste
- Fresh cilantro for garnish

INSTRUCTIONS

1. In a large bowl, combine shrimp, avocados, cherry tomatoes, and red onion.
2. In a small bowl, whisk together lime juice, olive oil, salt, and pepper. Pour over shrimp mixture and toss to coat.
3. Garnish with fresh cilantro before serving.

NUTRITIONAL FACTS

- Calories: 350
- Protein: 25g
- Carbohydrates: 10g
- Fat: 24g

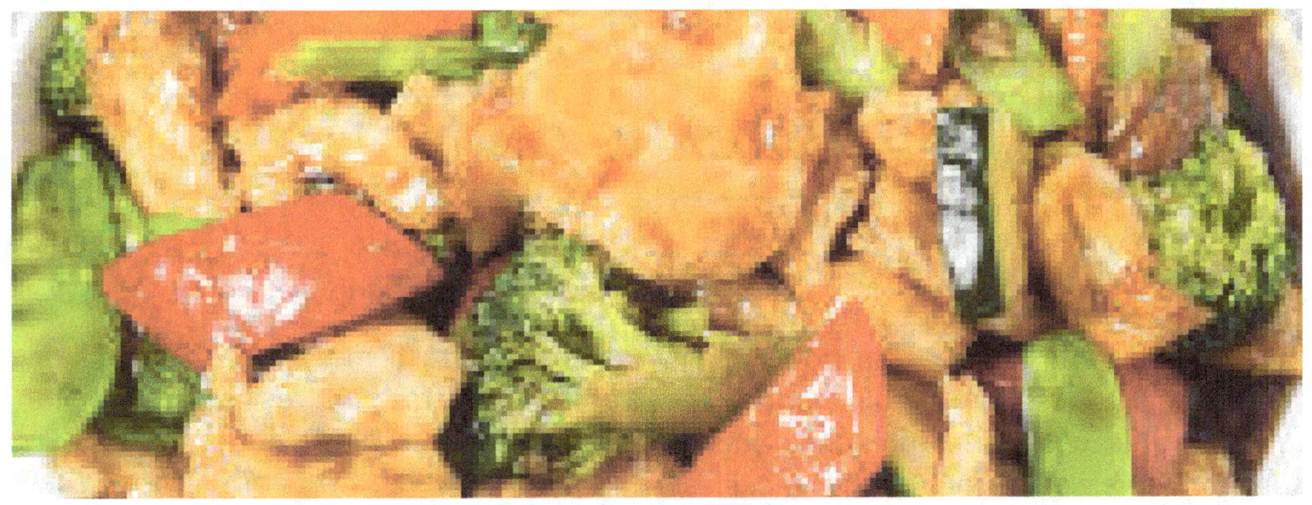

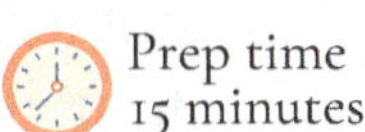 Prep time
15 minutes

 Cook time
15 minutes

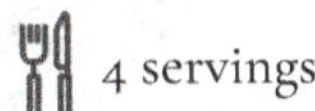 4 servings

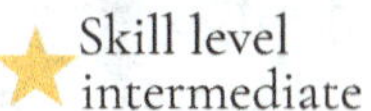 Skill level
intermediate

Chicken and Vegetable Stir-Fry

INGREDIENTS

ADDITIONAL

- 1 lb boneless, skinless chicken breast, thinly sliced
- 2 tablespoons soy sauce
- 1 tablespoon sesame oil
- 2 tablespoons olive oil
- 2 cups broccoli florets
- 1 red bell pepper, sliced
- 1 yellow bell pepper, sliced
- 1 carrot, julienned
- 3 cloves garlic, minced
- 1 tablespoon grated ginger
- 2 tablespoons hoisin sauce
- 2 tablespoons water
- 2 green onions, sliced
- Sesame seeds for garnish

INSTRUCTIONS

1. In a bowl, marinate chicken slices with soy sauce and sesame oil for 10 minutes.
2. Heat olive oil in a large skillet or wok over medium-high heat. Add chicken and cook until browned and cooked through. Remove from skillet and set aside.
3. In the same skillet, add broccoli, bell peppers, carrot, garlic, and ginger. Stir-fry for 5-7 minutes, or until vegetables are tender-crisp.
4. Return chicken to skillet. Add hoisin sauce and water, and stir to coat evenly.
5. Garnish with green onions and sesame seeds before serving.

NUTRITIONAL FACTS

- Calories: 300
- Protein: 30g
- Carbohydrates: 20g
- Fat: 12g

CONCLUSION

As we come to the end of this cookbook journey, I want to express my deepest gratitude to you, the readers, for joining me on this exploration of nutrition and its vital role in cancer care. Throughout these pages, we've delved into the complexities of nourishment during treatment, offering practical guidance, recipes, and meal plans designed to support your health and well-being.

Summary of Key Learnings

We've discussed the profound impact that thoughtful nutrition can have on your journey with cancer. From understanding the importance of balanced meals to discovering key nutrients that promote healing and strength, each chapter has been crafted with your health at its core.

Empowerment Through Nutrition

By embracing the recipes and meal plans provided in this cookbook, you've taken a proactive step towards nurturing your body and enhancing your quality of life. Food is not just sustenance but a powerful tool that empowers you to reclaim control and optimize your health during treatment

Encouragement and Support

Remember, each meal you prepare is an act of self-care and resilience. As you navigate the challenges of treatment, know that you are not alone. Your dedication to prioritizing nutrition is a testament to your strength and commitment to wellness.

Acknowledgment and Gratitude

I extend my heartfelt thanks to the healthcare professionals, researchers, and individuals who generously shared their expertise and experiences, making this cookbook possible. Your contributions have enriched the lives of countless individuals facing cancer.

Looking Ahead

As you continue your journey, I encourage you to explore further, experiment with new flavors, and adapt recipes to suit your preferences and nutritional needs. This cookbook is a starting point—a foundation upon which you can build a lifetime of healthy eating habits.

FINAL THOUGHTS

May this cookbook serve as a source of inspiration and practical support on your path to recovery and beyond. Your resilience and determination are a beacon of hope, and I am honored to have been a part of your journey towards better health.

NOTES

NOTES

NOTES